KU-370-598

LEARNING
to cope with
CRPS / RSD

*Putting life first and
pain second*

KAREN RODHAM

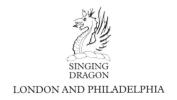

SINGING
DRAGON

LONDON AND PHILADELPHIA

The Four Pillars of Care (p.17), copyright © 2012 Royal College of Physicians, reproduced with permission from Goebel, A., Barker, C.H., Turner-Stokes, L. *et al.* (2012) *Complex Regional Pain Syndrome in Adults: UK Guidelines for Diagnosis, Referral and Management in Primary and Secondary Care.* London: RCP.

This edition published in 2015
by Singing Dragon
an imprint of Jessica Kingsley Publishers
73 Collier Street
London N1 9BE, UK
and
400 Market Street, Suite 400
Philadelphia, PA 19106, USA

www.singingdragon.com

First edition published by the author in 2013

Copyright © Karen Rodham 2013, 2015
Front cover image source: © Dengess | Dreamstime.com - Flowering Cactus Photo

All rights reserved. No part of this publication may be reproduced in any material form (including photocopying or storing it in any medium by electronic means and whether or not transiently or incidentally to some other use of this publication) without the written permission of the copyright owner except in accordance with the provisions of the Copyright, Designs and Patents Act 1988 or under the terms of a licence issued by the Copyright Licensing Agency Ltd, Saffron House, 6–10 Kirby Street, London EC1N 8TS. Applications for the copyright owner's written permission to reproduce any part of this publication should be addressed to the publisher.

Warning: The doing of an unauthorized act in relation to a copyright work may result in both a civil claim for damages and criminal prosecution.

Library of Congress Cataloging in Publication Data
Rodham, Karen, 1970-
  Learning to cope with CRSP/RSD : putting life first and CRPS/RSD second / Karen Rodham.
    pages cm
  Includes bibliographical references and index.
  ISBN 978-1-84819-240-9 (alk. paper)
  1. Reflex sympathetic dystrophy--Popular works. 2. Reflex sympathetic dystrophy--Patients--Biography. I. Title.
  RC422.R43R64 2015
  616'.0472--dc23

                          2014013397

British Library Cataloguing in Publication Data
A CIP catalogue record for this book is available from the British Library

ISBN 978 1 84819 240 9
eISBN 978 0 85701 188 6

Printed and bound in Great Britain

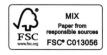

'Not in ten years…'
To all the Gadds and Gaddlets –
thank you for being you.

ACKNOWLEDGEMENTS

I'd like to take this opportunity to thank my colleagues (who are, truth be told, now friends too) at the Royal National Hospital for Rheumatic Diseases (RNHRD), with whom I have very much enjoyed working, and I'd also like to thank all the people living with CRPS who have shared their stories and experiences with me as we have worked together to find a way to cope with the challenges that come with CRPS; you have all taught me so much. Of course, I would also like to thank the RNHRD Donated Funds and Charitable Trustees Committee who funded the research that informs part of this book (Ref. RBB347). Lastly, thank you to Alison and to Julie who gave up their precious time to read and comment on earlier versions of this book.

CONTENTS

Introduction.   11

Chapter 1 What is CRPS?   13

Chapter 2 What is it like to live with CRPS?. . . .   23

    Happy *58, male – left hand and wrist*   26

    Helen *44, female – left arm, left leg, back*.   32

    Cloggy *56, female – left arm, left shoulder, neck*.   38

    Sam *46, male – left side of head, left arm, left leg*   45

    Sarah *48, female – left leg*   52

    Melanie *48, female – left leg*.   59

    Thomas *30, male – right leg, both arms*.   66

    Crystal *44, female – right arm, both shoulders,*
       left leg.   72

    Stella *65, female – left arm*   79

    Snoopy *46, female – both legs*.   86

Chapter 3 How can I cope with CRPS?.   93

Chapter 4 CRPS does not just affect the person
who is diagnosed with CRPS 121

Chapter 5 Endings 131

USEFUL RESOURCES 133

REFERENCES 139

INDEX 141

INTRODUCTION

In the UK we use the term Complex Regional Pain Syndrome (CRPS), but in America, it is more common to use the term RSD (Reflex Sympathetic Dystrophy). Throughout this book, I will be using the UK term CRPS.

If you are reading this book, I imagine you are either living with CRPS yourself or know someone who has the condition. This book is something I have wanted to write for a while. I have been working with people living with the chronic form of CRPS since 2006 and now feel as if I have enough of an insight into this 'difficult-to-live-with' condition to share the lessons I have learned from the people I have worked with.

It is my hope that this book will be useful to those who are themselves living with chronic CRPS, because within its the pages they will see that they are not alone. I also hope it will be a useful resource for friends, family and colleagues of people living with CRPS, because it will enable them to have a glimpse of what it is like to live with CRPS. Through this glimpse, their understanding will grow and their ability to support the person who has CRPS will grow too.

I have also written this book as a last offering in my role as CRPS Health Psychologist, for I will be leaving the 'Min' shortly after this book is published and I wanted to make sure that the knowledge I have been privileged to gain over the past seven or so years is presented in book form so that other psychologists can build on the lessons I have learned, and, perhaps most importantly, I hope that people living with CRPS and their friends and family will find the content useful.

Chapter 1

WHAT IS CRPS?

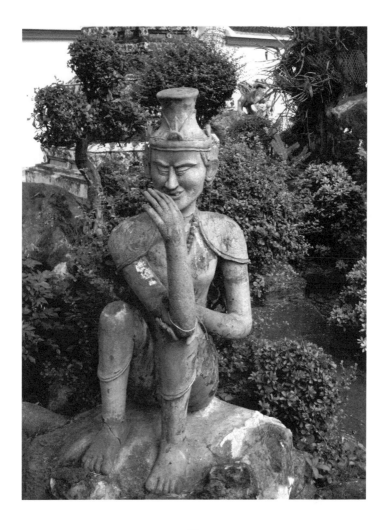

Complex Regional Pain Syndrome (CRPS) is a pain condition that usually occurs after an injury, but it can start spontaneously (Harden *et al.* 2010; Kozin 2005; McBride and Atkins 2005; Stanton-Hicks 2006). Burning pain is the most characteristic symptom, but people also report swelling, coldness, colour changes, hypersensitivity, as well as increased sweat and hair growth. A person who is herself living with CRPS, who very kindly read a draft of this book, told me that although the original description of the symptoms that I had included was technically correct, she felt it downplayed the experience of pain. To her, CRPS was 'pain, pain, pain'. I promised to include her quote to make sure that this was absolutely clear. Although the symptoms are *usually* experienced in a single limb, it is possible for CRPS to occur in more than one limb, and indeed in other body regions (Baron *et al.* 2002; Galer *et al.* 2000; Kozin 2005; Stanton-Hicks *et al.* 1995; Veldman *et al.* 1993). For an estimated 7 per cent of people, CRPS can spread to other limbs.

Many people who have CRPS experience it as a transient problem. De Mos and colleagues (2009) suggest that about 85 per cent of people improve within the first year after onset, but Goebel and colleagues (2012) point out that it is important to remember that improvement does not necessarily equal recovery. Indeed, they go on to say that a definition of what constitutes recovery has not yet been agreed. It might be more accurate to say that, rather than the symptoms disappearing, improvement means that people have found a way to live with the symptoms. So, there is a significant minority of people (about 15–20%) who will develop chronic CRPS. For this group of people, the experience of long-term symptoms or impairment is common. It is this group of people that I have worked with since 2006, and it is this group – who are essentially living with a long-term chronic pain condition – that this book is directed at.

DIAGNOSIS

Diagnosis is based on the Budapest Criteria, drawn up by an international group of CRPS experts to help health professionals make a diagnosis. These have now been adopted by the International Association for the Study of Pain (IASP) and can also be found on the website of Royal College of Physicians. Whilst these criteria are undoubtedly useful, one challenge for health professionals looking to explain a patient's symptoms is that there are currently no tests or biomarkers to confirm diagnosis of CRPS. So, while prompt diagnosis combined with early treatment is recommended, it is not so straightforward. CRPS is not a common condition and, as such, few health professionals will be familiar with it. Add to this the many names that CRPS has had in the past – Algodystrophy, Sudeck's Atrophy, Causalgia, Reflex Sympathetic Dystrophy, Shoulder-Hand Syndrome, Fracture Disease – and if you also consider the problem that the range of CRPS symptoms could be signs of a large number of other serious conditions, it can take some time for other possible explanations to be ruled out. This means that people with CRPS often experience a series of different (mis)diagnoses and a consequent delay in diagnosing CRPS.

Indeed, for many of the people I have worked with, the process of receiving a formal diagnosis has been a lengthy one. The uncertainty that surrounds this process can be very unsettling for the person concerned and may result in them questioning whether their symptoms are 'all in their mind' when test results are repeatedly negative and healthcare professionals seem unsure about how to explain their symptoms. As a result, when a person receives their diagnosis, this can be a mixed blessing: there is finally an explanation for their symptoms, but there remains uncertainty about prognosis, mixed with frustration at the length of time it has taken to reach a diagnosis.

HOW IS CRPS TREATED?

The 'Gold Standard' for treating CRPS conforms to the Four Pillars of Care (see Figure 1.1). These aim to reduce pain, restore function, enable people to manage their condition and improve their quality of life (Harden 2001).

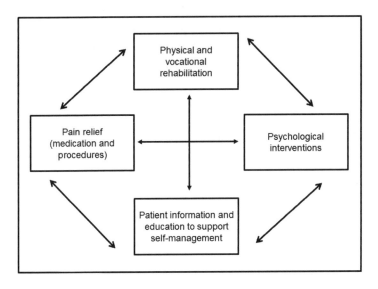

Figure 1.1: The Four Pillars of Care
Reproduced from Goebel, A., Barker, C.H., Turner-Stokes, L. *et al.* (2012)
Complex Regional Pain Syndrome in Adults: UK Guidelines for Diagnosis,
Referral and Management in Primary and Secondary Care. London: RCP.

Pain relief

The majority of people living with CRPS with whom I have worked tell me that the best the medication does is to take the edge off their pain. For some, there are problems related to the side effects of the medication, including drowsiness – sometimes to the point that they find it difficult to function. I have heard pain specialists speak at conferences about pain medication; they often call it a process of trial and error. This can be very frustrating for the person with CRPS because it can take some time to find a combination of medication that works for them. Sometimes, after all this, the person with CRPS decides to learn to manage without taking any medication because the negative impact of the side effects outweighs the positive impact of the slight pain reduction. Whatever your decision, be sure to talk it over with a doctor who is a pain specialist; they will be able to advise you of the pros and cons of each type of pain medication you are considering and will work with you to make a decision about what is best for you.

Physical and vocational rehabilitation

Physical and vocational rehabilitation delivered by experienced physiotherapists and occupational therapists is essential. This is because it can help people to regain or retain function. Key here is the idea that people with CRPS must play an active role. It is certainly not about a person having exercises *done* to them, but it *is* of paramount importance that the person with CRPS learns how to do the exercises themselves *and* finds the motivation to continue the exercises without the therapist being present. The person with CRPS needs to be willing to take control and responsibility so that they can become an active manager of their condition.

Physiotherapists and occupational therapists with expertise in CRPS will have been trained in CRPS-specific treatment approaches, which can include desensitization, mirror therapy and graded motor imagery. They can also work with those people who have body perception disturbance, also known as BPD (Lewis *et al.* 2007). Those who have BPD may perceive their affected limb as being grossly swollen and/or ugly; in some cases, part of their affected limb seems to them to have disappeared. This is obviously very upsetting to experience, and the therapists can work with a variety of techniques to help 'retune' the perceptions held by the person with CRPS.

Psychological interventions

Many people with CRPS are nervous about seeing psychologists. This is often because, at some point in their journey to diagnosis, someone somewhere may well have suggested to them that their pain is *all in their head* – or, in other words, is psychosomatic. They may well be afraid of seeing a psychologist because they fear that the appointment has been made for them by someone who does not believe they have CRPS.

Both researchers and clinicians are agreed that there is a reciprocal relationship between pain and psychosocial factors. So, although the notion that CRPS might be triggered by psychosocial factors is not fully supported by the research, the fact that CRPS can bring with it psychosocial problems has been clearly demonstrated (these problems include anxiety, depression, reduced quality of life, functional and occupational disability). This makes the role of psychologists important and a key part of a multidisciplinary team (Lohnberg and Altmaier 2013).

Indeed, the first job for the psychologist when meeting someone with CRPS is to reassure them that their CRPS is real and that they are not imagining their symptoms. The role of the psychologist is very much focused on finding out how the person with CRPS is coping, and on using the theories and strategies from psychology to help the person to cope better. Common issues that psychologists will cover include:

- Loss: loss of identity, loss of self-esteem, loss of hobbies, loss of role, loss of independence, loss of job, loss of social life, loss of intimacy.

- Communication: explaining CRPS to others, asking for help when you are the person who always used to give help, dealing with other people's inappropriate questions.

- Stress management: dealing with negative thoughts, coping with anxiety about the treatment, relaxation strategies, fear of going out, fear of being bumped.

- Goal setting: working out how to set goals, how to make sure goals are realistic, how to pace when working towards goals.

Ideally, psychologists should work closely with the physical therapists to make sure that psychological therapy is integrated with the treatment programme. In this way, the psychological coping techniques can be both supported and reinforced by the physical therapists.

Patient information and education

Of course, it is really important for you to find out as much as you can about CRPS. This might be easier said than done, especially if you are searching the internet. There is a lot of unsubstantiated information out there in cyberspace, much of which is frightening. You are probably familiar with the saying 'forewarned is forearmed' and I agree that it is good to find out what you can about CRPS, but I also think that you should do so with the following in mind. There seems to be no clear route for the progression of CRPS, so just because one person has experienced symptoms, or has found that their CRPS has spread, this does not mean that this is what is in store for you too. A good strategy would be to talk with your therapists and ask them which websites and sources of information they would recommend.

Another thing that people with CRPS tell me is that they struggle to get hold of academic papers that have been published. It can be expensive to buy the papers. A top tip from me (I am an academic as well as a psychologist) would be to email the main author of the paper and ask them if you could have a copy. Sometimes, if copyright allows, we have permission to send copies of our papers to those who contact us.

So, now you have a brief explanation of what CRPS is, how it is diagnosed and treated. But in order to bring the actual experience of what it is *like* to have CRPS, it is important to hear the voices of those who have been living with the condition; after all, they are the ones who *really* know what it is like. The next chapter presents ten people's stories.

Chapter 2

WHAT IS IT LIKE TO LIVE WITH CRPS?

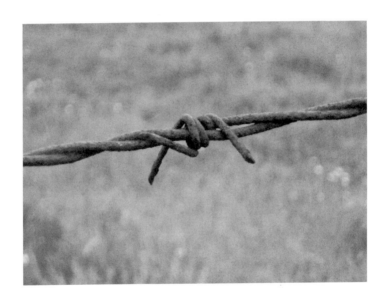

In this chapter we look at ten people's stories. I have chosen them at random from a range of interviews I completed for different research projects. Each interview lasted about an hour and produced around 50 pages of typed conversation. It would be far too overwhelming to include all that detail, so I have turned each interview into a mini case study. Each person tells their story, focusing on how CRPS has impacted on them and how they have tried to cope. Their names and the names of other people and places mentioned are disguised to protect each person's identity. I have used direct quotes from the interviews so that you can almost hear each person's voice. The quotes include the 'erms' and 'ums'. Sometimes you will see [...] which means I have taken out a section of the interview that was not directly relevant to the point being made.

Inevitably, these stories just provide a snapshot and show how different people have reacted to, and coped with, the challenges that come when living with chronic CRPS. My hope is that reading these people's stories will show you that you are not alone and that others have also experienced similar battles to those you are currently fighting.

One other thing: each person I interviewed was invited to choose the name they wanted to be used in the write-up. This is why some of the stories are from people called Happy, Snoopy and Cloggy.

HAPPY

*'So I went down, cap-in-hand to my doctor, my
GP, and I said I've been diagnosed, I've got a
preliminary diagnosis of CRPS. They think I've
got CRPS and they want me to get it checked
out. And he said, "Er. Pardon. What's that?"'*

Happy chose this pseudonym because he felt it best
reflected his approach to life. He was 58 years old at the
time of the interview. He had been diagnosed for one year
and had CRPS in his left hand and wrist. He lived at home
with his wife and adult daughter. Happy's CRPS began when
he had a 'contracture' (a permanent shortening of the muscle
or tendon) in his hand. After an operation, Happy was put in
a cast which he found excruciatingly painful. He said that
it took about three months for CRPS to be suspected. Until
then, his hand therapist continued normal hand therapy –
this involved manipulating Happy's fingers which was very
difficult for him to tolerate:

> *Bless her, she actually asked me to sit on the other hand
> once because she thought I was going to hit her! [...]
> actively like bending my fingers straight, trying and then
> forcing my hand into a fist and it was just excruciating.*

The senior hand therapist noticed that Happy's hand was
changing colour, mottling and swelling, and suggested that
he might have CRPS. This was the first time he had heard of
the condition. The hand therapy team tried to explain what
CRPS was, but he found it difficult to understand. They also
prescribed medication to help with the pain:

They explained it like that it was this vicious circle that the hand was broken somewhere so they put me on some really heavy stuff, erm, er, that I was on loads and loads of tablets all day and I couldn't hardly think straight [...] I wouldn't even be able to talk to anyone before half past eleven in the morning. It was hopeless. Anything anyone said to me I didn't remember and it was just like being a zombie really and it was awful.

So the medication had a really negative impact on his ability to function normally. In addition, he said that the hand therapists referred him back to his surgeon once they suspected CRPS, but he felt that his surgeon then engaged in what he called a 'blaming-game', laying the blame for his problems at the therapist's door:

So as soon as they thought this might be CRPS, they, erm, they contacted my surgeon again because he kept saying, (the surgeon who did the operation), kept saying that it's the hand therapists; they're not doing their job and that's why it's not working, and all these things. [...] So, erm, he was blaming the hand therapist.

Being stuck in the middle of this 'blame game' was a really uncomfortable place to be and it was not helping Happy at all. Happy had read about the CRPS service at Bath and made an appointment with his GP (family doctor) to try to convince him to make a referral to Bath, but during his appointment it became apparent that his GP had not heard of CRPS:

So I went down, cap-in-hand to my doctor, my GP, and I said I've been diagnosed, I've got a preliminary diagnosis of CRPS. They think I've got CRPS and they want me to get it checked out. And he said, 'Er. Pardon. What's that?'

Happy's heart must have really sunk at this response. He was now in a position where he felt that he had to take control and responsibility for convincing the health profession to refer him. His doctor asked him to leave it for the weekend and to come back the following week. This was a low moment, but when they met again:

> *He'd been on the internet; he'd written to his people, I think he might have written to your people in Bath, he'd written to everybody, and he was so helpful. He was so helpful, my GP. And he really sort of pushed and pushed to get me on the programme.*

This was a huge relief because searching the internet for CRPS-related information had been a frightening experience and, at the same time, Happy was struggling with the side effects of the pain medication, changes in his visual perception and fear that someone might bump into his painful hand:

> *Everything was crazy. All of a sudden I'd be trying to, erm, in the afternoons when the drugs had worn off a bit, trying to read a book or watch television and everything started moving about. Erm. Words were jumping off the page and the television was shaking and shivering. It wasn't, I know it wasn't, and, erm, you are walking around, I was walking around with my hand on the bottom, by the bottom of my neck, centre of my chest to try and keep it, erm, protected. So everything, everything about my life, really sounds a bit trivial what I just said, but everything, everything was affected. I was severely, um, miserable.*

He was also struggling with a change in his identity:

> *Frustrating to the nth degree, especially when you have been an active sort of person. Frustrating. It is depressing, it's erm, exhausting being in pain all day, is absolutely exhausting. It wears you right out.*

In particular, the fact that no one could see the pain he was experiencing was incredibly frustrating; he felt that it made it difficult for them to understand what he was going through:

> All you've got is like a slightly, erm to them, slightly mottled wax-works looking hand [...]. It is waxy and this funny mottly colour and that's, that's the only outward sign to anyone else and they think, 'Well, what's up with you? Why are you making such a bloody fuss?'

Happy thought his hand looked alien and much larger than his non-affected hand:

> It looked completely alien [...] or something like, erm, I have described it as a baseball catcher's mitt. That's what it looked like to me. It was huge. It was just so, erm, I don't know. Well, it appeared enormous. And there was, it was more like a mitten than a hand. There was a thumb, but there were...the fingers just merged into one another.

Experiencing his hand in this way, whilst knowing that to others it looked relatively normal, was a challenge to his sense of self. He felt at times as if he was 'going stupid, going doolally. It almost makes you convince yourself that you are going insane.' So, on one level, Happy was aware of the symptoms that accompanied CRPS and knew that they were real, but, on another level, he doubted his sanity because his perception of his hand was so skewed.

At the time of the interview, Happy felt that he was coping well and that he was making good headway on learning to live with CRPS: 'I've learned not to control it, but to live with it a bit.' Completing the rehabilitation programme equipped him with a set of tools he could use and raised his awareness of the subtle ways in which CRPS had begun to affect him:

There were lots of things happening that I was not aware of. Things like, I didn't know where my hand was when I couldn't see it. I had no perception, I wasn't spatially aware of where my hand was. As soon as it went outside of vision, it could have been anywhere, erm, and I realized I have been cheating really, because I know that my hand therapist said that she'd been reading books and that you've got to love your, love your hand. You've got to keep looking at it and do this and everything else. I'm not pooh-poohing what she said, it's good advice, but I admit that when I was at the hospital I realized that I'd been cheating.

Being challenged by the team helped him to recognize the often unconscious coping strategies he had adopted, and allowed him to undo them and replace them with more helpful coping strategies. Initially, Happy had been resistant to accepting CRPS, but he came to realize that 'by accepting it you can, that's the only way you can start to try to make things better'. Working towards his own acceptance was hard enough in itself, but it was exponentially harder when members of the health profession did not believe in CRPS:

They just do not believe that you are in pain. They just can't see it. There's nothing. The pain is so disproportionate if you like, to the, to the actual physical symptoms, that they think, 'What are you playing at?' and sometimes you want to walk around with a plaque on saying, 'I'm in real pain here, please leave me alone' [laughs].

Having to explain CRPS to health professionals, who are gatekeepers to treatment, and feeling that he had to justify why he needed more medication was exhausting. As such, his key message for coping was to be sure to inform yourself about CRPS by finding 'good quality information that is presented in a way that is not alarming'. He was very clear that people with CRPS needed to know that they were not alone and that there was help out there. Attending the rehabilitation programme had really helped him to come to terms with his diagnosis; as his understanding of the condition grew, so did his acceptance and his ability to cope. It also helped him to realize he was not alone:

> So I know I'm not unique in it, and you know, you know I've begun to feel a bit grateful really 'cos I'm, I consider myself, I've got a very mild form of it, I think.

In sum, Happy felt that he had made good progress. He was learning to live with CRPS and was focusing on the positive. This was reflected in the pseudonym that he chose for himself. He did not shy away from talking about his negative experiences, but his interview was marked throughout by his explicit and active attempts to look for the positive in all he did.

HELEN

*'I think everybody, or a lot of people with CRPS, will
all say the same, that they've lost their circle of
friends. There'll be so many people that will go, you
know, back away from you, and I think it is natural
because you back away and they do the same.'*

Helen was 44 years old and married at the time of the
interview. She had been diagnosed for one and a half
years and had CRPS in her left arm and leg, and in most of
her back. Her CRPS began immediately following a traffic
accident:

> *I was sat waiting to go out of the junction and a car came
> down a slip road and decided it had enough time to cut
> across oncoming traffic, and didn't. And, uh, he ended up
> in the side of me. Um, and straight away my arm was in
> agony. And it's never gone away.*

Shortly after the accident, Helen said that CRPS was
mentioned in passing as a possibility, but no one explained
to her what this might mean. Things then became
complicated because her car insurance company took
control and told her that they would get her all the medical
help and rehabilitation she needed. She talked things over
with her GP who thought that going through the insurance
company would probably 'fast-track' her. However:

> *So I was, um, now I know, stupid enough to go along with
> this because I believed what they said. And I was with
> them [insurance company] for about 14 months...and all
> they did in that time, was they, they actually sent me for*

what I was told was a rehabilitation appointment but it wasn't. It was for court evidence. And, um, sent me for an MRI scan and also recommended that I had a visit to the pain, er, pain clinic. But they never set me up an appointment. And I was chasing and chasing them all the time. Kept going back to my GP and she was saying, 'Well, you know you're still in the best of hands, because you've still got the barrier of the 12–18 month [NHS] waiting list.' Um, so basically after about 15 months when nothing was happening... Well in the October afterwards, um, October 2007, they came back to me and said it was, that I was mental. That is was all in my head. That there was nothing wrong with me and I needed psychiatric help and basically go away and leave us alone. Which I took quite hard at the time, um, because obviously you question yourself to think: Well, is it me?

Helen had therefore had a long wait and received mixed and unclear messages. What she was expecting from the insurance company was not what was delivered; she was not offered treatment and said that she was accused of having a psychological problem. Not surprisingly, Helen began to doubt herself. She began to see other specialists who she said were none the wiser and just as doubtful about her symptoms:

People were, you know, saying, 'Well, it should have been better by now', um, you know, so I had lots and lots of little bits of people not believing me. You know, which gets you a wee bit down as well because you're sort of thinking 'Well, I'm in pain' and, you know, you get treated for depression, but that's not the problem.

So Helen really struggled to get a clear diagnosis that actually explained her symptoms. She kept being told that she would or should 'be better' in a few weeks' time. The ever-changing goalposts were frustrating and exhausting and difficult to cope with. Helen had also just started a new business and was extremely concerned about the impact her symptoms might have:

> I just thought, you know, we have invested a huge amount of money in this, and you know, all my family's confidence and everything, you know, backing me.

Helen tried to carry on and ignore the pain she was experiencing, but eventually she reluctantly closed her business. The combination of the increase in her pain, the spread of her symptoms down her shoulder and into her back, and her inability to continue running her business led her to fear what might be wrong. Several worst-case scenarios were running through her mind. She began to push her GP to refer her for further help and eventually one of the people conducting an ultrasound mentioned CRPS and Helen asked to be referred to Bath.

As she spoke, her relief at coming to the rehabilitation programme was tangible. She felt that she began to understand CRPS and said that she learned different coping strategies. However, knowing about good coping strategies and putting them into practice are very different things. Pacing in particular was a strategy she struggled with and was for her a compromise that involved changing the way she thought about how things should be:

> The reality of doing that [pacing] is, um, you know, the house doesn't get hoovered, and, um, you know...yeah, there's a compromise, yeah. And that's hard for somebody like me who's very much a perfectionist.

Helen spoke about the difficult transition from busy and independent businesswoman to someone who needed to pace herself. Looking back, she found it hard to see how she had ever managed to fit everything into her life before

CRPS and could no longer recognize her current self in the 'person' she once was:

> You know, I can't equate myself with being that person that I was, which may sound strange [laughs] but you know, um, you know...

There was a sense of grief for the things she had lost. She was no longer able to go walking or cycling, and she recognized with hindsight that for a time she had been on a 'downward spiral' and had become passive: someone who waited to be asked to do things, rather than instigating things. She had become a person who had retreated into her house. She recognized that completing the rehabilitation programme had helped her to 'refocus'. By this, she meant that she began to turn her thinking around from being inward-focused to more outward-focused.

Meeting other people with CRPS who were also on the programme was an incredibly positive experience for Helen. They kept in touch and formed an informal support group on their return home. This was especially important because she had noticed that some of her 'pre-CRPS' friends had backed away:

> I think everybody, or a lot of people with CRPS, will all say the same, that they've lost their circle of friends. There'll be so many people that will go, you know, back away from you, and I think it is mutual because you back away and they do the same.

This quote highlights a tricky issue. Many friends are uncertain about how to help and, in their embarrassment, back away. Similarly, people living with CRPS often talk about feeling that they have become a burden, and they too back away. So, at a time when support is really important, the support network can reduce, often because neither party can find a way of communicating how they are feeling.

A further benefit of having friends who themselves had CRPS was the ability to share how she was really feeling without being afraid of worrying them in the way that family would be worried:

> Um, if you say, 'No, I've had a really bad night. I've not slept for two days, you know, I'm in so much pain I don't want to be here' or something like that, people [with CRPS] understand you. And it is not that you actually don't want to be here, it's just that, it's being allowed to say that sometimes, without causing alarm bells, I think. Because, it's, because other people would find that, um, I think family find it distressing.

It was really important for Helen to feel she was regaining some of the control that she felt she had lost as a consequence of the CRPS. Finding ways to do this took time. Things that worked well for Helen included writing down her feelings in what she described as 'scribbles and poems', as well as practising mindfulness and being completely in the present moment:

> If I'm feeling very down, I'll go and think, well OK, I'm gonna go out in the garden for 5 minutes or, I'm going to totally, um, take my mind off it.

In terms of issues that interfered with Helen's ability to cope, a major one concerned the court case and related litigation that was ongoing at the time of the interview. Helen was aware that 'the other side' had had her under surveillance, which she had naturally found very uncomfortable because it was another example of someone not believing that she had CRPS as well as not understanding the unpredictability of CRPS:

> I've been, you know, had surveillance done of me, which I find very difficult, the fact that I am being watched, um,

when I have done nothing wrong. You know, I'd like to go back where I, you know, four and a half years ago and not have been at that junction and not be like I am now.

Dealing with this was difficult and frustrating. Helen described the process as being '*a game to them, and it's not. It's my life.*' She felt that the important issue should have been *her*, and the impact on *her life*, but somehow this was lost in all the legal games that were being 'played'.

CLOGGY

'The relief. It was a relief. Ahh. It is NOT in my
mind. There IS something there. And once I had a
diagnosis it is as if a light bulb went on and I thought,
"Ah. Now I know what it is, I can cope with it."'

Cloggy was 56 years old at the time of the interview. She had
been diagnosed for two and a half years. She had CRPS in
her left arm, shoulder and neck. She lived with her husband.
Her CRPS had started gradually; she said that her job at the
time had involved lots of computer work and she began
to get an ache in her shoulder. She ignored this for some
time, but then began to get other symptoms in her fingers.
She ignored these symptoms too, rationalizing them away.
These symptoms went on for a year, and suddenly, whilst at
her workstation, she experienced a wave of pain:

> I noticed I was getting an ache in the shoulder, and I
> wasn't sure what it was, so I, um, like everything else, you
> just put it to the back of your mind and get on with it.
> You know, you just... Then I started getting tingling in my
> fingers and I was just thinking I have been lying wrong
> in bed, you know? Because it was usually in the morning.
> And, um, we'd been on holiday and we'd come back and
> I went to do some work on the computer and my hand's
> always stuck in the same position, so caught between a
> keyboard, and something went 'woof' in my shoulder. Oh!
> The pain. I actually had tears in my eyes immediately, so
> I knew something was wrong.

Cloggy said that she spent a year trying to explain away the symptoms she had been experiencing, but once the pain arrived, she went straight to her GP. The GP sent her for ten sessions of physiotherapy, which had no effect. She also saw an orthopaedic surgeon, who carried out a number of tests (MRI scans, nerve conduction, ultrasound) and she was diagnosed with bursitis. (NHS Direct defines bursitis as inflammation and swelling of a bursa. A bursa is a fluid-filled sac which forms under the skin, usually over the joints and acts as a cushion between the tendons and bones.) She was given steroid injections which had no impact. She then had surgery, which also had no impact. Cloggy said that the pain was getting progressively worse and she still had no answers.

Cloggy returned to work on a part-time basis, but the pain was difficult to cope with and she returned many times to her GP, who referred her to a pain clinic. At this clinic she said she was given a leaflet, but nothing was explained to her. She was also told to return to work on a full-time basis. She struggled and although her employer made some adjustments, the pain was awful, and she began to think it must be in her mind: 'And in the end, I admit I was thinking "Oh, it is just in your mind half the time."' She returned to her orthopaedic surgeon who did a further procedure, following which her pain increased dramatically and her hand began to alter:

> And then after that it just went 'woof' completely off the scale. My fingers started to turn in. Um, oh, the pain was horrendous. So the pain clinic opted, they sort of kept pushing my pain medication up.

After this, Cloggy said she was referred to a rheumatologist who diagnosed CRPS. So, from her first experience of pain to diagnosis took three years. Throughout that time she was veering between assuming that the aches and pains she was experiencing were perhaps a normal part of the ageing process and being afraid that the pains were a sign of something serious:

> Deep in my mind, I thought, oh, it is just old age. You know when you put things down, you've got a niggle, you've got a pain... And I never, you know, like I said, at some stage, I just thought, am I imagining this? Is it not as bad as I am thinking? But I mean, I was coming home after a full day's work, I was just sitting there crying.

This level of doubt and uncertainty also led Cloggy to imagine worst-case scenarios, which she then looked up on the internet. She mentioned becoming fearful that she might have multiple sclerosis and explained that she came to realize that searching for information on the internet was not at all helpful and actually fed her fears: 'You know, the internet doesn't help either. 'Cos you look things up and think "Oh God!"'

Coping with the pain, along with the uncertainty over diagnosis for those three years, was very difficult. Cloggy spoke of her fear that others would assume that she was making up her symptoms: 'It was quite hard to cope with because I'm also thinking about the people around me. What if they are thinking I am putting it on?'

When Cloggy got a diagnosis of CRPS, she said it was a huge relief and reassuring to be told by someone in authority that what she had was real. Being given a name for what she was experiencing immediately gave her confidence that she could deal with it:

> The relief. It was a relief. Ahh. It is NOT in my mind. There IS something there. And once I had a diagnosis, it is as if a lightbulb went on and I thought, 'Ah. Now I know what it is, I can cope with it.'

The label meant that she could look more efficiently for information (Cloggy's way of coping was to arm herself with knowledge); in so doing, she was increasing her confidence in her ability to take control and to actively cope:

> Once I knew what it was, I looked it up. I'd got all the reading material and I thought, 'OK, I can cope with this. I'm strong enough.'

Although she was keen to return to work on a part-time basis if adjustments were made to her role and her workstation, she suspects that her employers were not willing to do these things and as a consequence she lost her job. She spoke about this period in a very matter-of-fact tone, but when we discussed it further it was clear that she had been very hurt by this experience, and by the realization that her work friends were colleagues, not friends (once she became ill, they did not keep in touch). She said that she had felt very rejected and upset that she had given many years and worked hard for the company, and yet she feels she received so little in return.

> They weren't friends. They were work mates, which I thought were friends. They'd stopped; when I was ill, they stopped.

Cloggy spoke of having a difficult time coming to terms with the changes that had been imposed on her because of the CRPS. She said that she developed panic attacks and isolated herself for a couple of months:

> Um, I just didn't want to meet people. Uh. Dunno. It's just [...] all I did for a couple of months is sit on a sofa, watch TV.

She described a couple of unpleasant experiences that had happened when she was in town and people had bumped into her. For a while afterwards, she became afraid of busy, noisy places and noticed that she was monitoring everybody around her to make sure that they were not going to come near her. She would only go to places that she knew would be quiet and relatively empty. The more isolated she became, the more time she had to brood on CRPS and how her life had changed. She described this as a 'dark time'. It was then that she took up embroidery. Although she could not do it for lengthy periods, she found that she could 'lose herself' in the sewing and so 'escape' for a short while:

> It sort of took me away. It's... It's... It just...it stopped me thinking and that's what a lot of this is. If you've got nothing to do, you think constantly about pain.

Trying to explain CRPS to others has been tricky, to say the least. Other people don't understand it, and Cloggy herself recognizes how difficult it is to understand, and so she took to telling people that she had a 'rare form of arthritis'. She found that people understood this explanation, and recognized that arthritis was long-term, not necessarily visible and painful. Cloggy also found that trying to explain CRPS to others in terms of the nervous system and the brain almost always led them to think, 'Is she mental?'

However, Cloggy was not one to dwell on the negative side of things. She said that she got angry and then let her negative feelings go ('And then I thought "Oh, sod you!"'). She sought out a new job. At the time of the interview, she was working 14 hours a week over three days and was really enjoying it. Armed with the knowledge that work colleagues are not necessarily friends, she had become very boundaried:

> And now I'm in a new job I'm very careful not to make that mistake again. Friends at work, no. Outside of work, that's it.

Cloggy searched for other things that she could do and sought out new activities and interests, including going to the gym three or four times a week, swimming and short courses. It was not an easy process and involved a lot of trial and error before she found things she could manage. The key was in not giving up:

> I tried all the classes, I tied pilates, yoga, tai chi. Pilates and yoga were too strenuous, you know, because there is a lot of groundwork and I couldn't put my arm down, so I stuck with tai chi.

She also actively reduced the medication she was taking: '*I think I've taken too many drugs over the years and I don't like it and I'm slowly reducing it.*' She took the decision that CRPS was a thing to be battled, and this was how she framed her coping strategies. She was very clear, though, that before you could battle the condition, you had to accept it:

> If you don't accept it, how can you fight against something that you don't accept?

She also spoke of the importance of listening to and following the advice of the health professionals with CRPS expertise:

> They don't tell you 'don't do this' just for the fun of it. They have been working with people for a long, long time. They know what they are talking about.

At the time of the interview, Cloggy was feeling that she was more in control and accepting of CRPS. She was holding down a job that she enjoyed and continuing her exercises, and she felt as though she was on an upward trajectory: '*I'm not back to the same person I was before, but I am getting there.*' She was remaining positive in outlook and recognized the importance of not putting every ache and pain down to CRPS. She was aware that it would be easy to blame CRPS for everything, and she was mindful of this temptation and resisted it:

> It's intertwined, 'cos, you know, I can blame everything on CRPS, but it is not always CRPS. It's also, like I said, the ageing process. It's sort of...more tired – is it because of the drugs, the CRPS, or it is just old age?

In short, for Cloggy, fighting CRPS was the key and her take-home message was 'never give up'.

SAM

'I feel like Dracula sometimes because sunlight can come through the window and the heat from the sunlight (I just keep my feet off). It can set it off. I can feel it radiating out and I'm bursting into flames in my foot.'

Sam was 46 years old at the time of the interview and he had been diagnosed for two years. Following a workplace injury, he developed CRPS on the left side of his head, in his left arm and in his left leg. He had assumed his injury would heal, but it just 'got worse and worse'. As a consequence, the healthcare profession began to search for an explanation for his symptoms:

> *Started up having investigations...nobody really knew what was going on. They said, 'Oh yeah, it'll heal up in six months, and then twelve months.' Erm, the injury did heal itself...the broken bones, that was fine. Then it was just the pain and the burning pain and the things going on inside my head basically.*

What was confusing for Sam was the idea that although the original injury *had* healed, he was not getting better; he was still in pain, he said his head did not seem to be able to recognize his foot, and in addition to the pain and the swelling, Sam was aware of strange perceptual things going on. For example, he felt that the CRPS-affected parts of his body were enormously swollen, even though friends and family were telling him otherwise. He also found he was greatly sensitive to touch and was unable to wear shoes for a while, because his foot would not tolerate them:

> I had to have my shoes off, you know... I can't wear anything tight, I can't even do my shoelace up tight because that's, you know, it's the movement of it dug into me really...erm, and it [CRPS] sort of spread from my foot up my leg just below my knee, and then I had it in my face and my head... Of course, I was thinking that my face was out here [indicates with his hand how swollen he perceived his face to be], and my brain was telling me nothing...

One of the most frustrating things for Sam – in fact the first issue he raised just as the interview was getting started – was about the lack of understanding he had encountered from everyone around him – professionals and lay people alike. This lack of understanding, particularly from the health profession, caused Sam to doubt them *and* himself:

> Other people, I found, didn't understand what was going on. People I was seeing didn't really know what was going on, erm. So you didn't have faith in them and you didn't have faith in yourself because you couldn't believe it yourself.

He was sent for a number of what were, for him, frightening tests, because he was aware that the symptoms he was experiencing could have also been the result of a stroke. He was therefore imagining worst-case scenarios. As a consequence, when each test result was negative, Sam felt a mixture of relief that a particular issue had been ruled out and fear that, because there was still no explanation for his symptoms, an alternative worst-case scenario might explain them. In short, his symptoms were unexplained and were therefore still something to worry about. Sam said it took about two years following the accident to be referred to a pain management team. At this point, the diagnosis of RSD was being talked about:

> *Somebody picked up on, well they used to call it RSD, wasn't it? Yes, so somebody knew it was probably RSD. Course, it didn't mean anything to me [laughs] 'cos I'd never heard of it.*

Sam worked with the pain management team who explained that RSD was now called CRPS, and they focused on *'attacking that with tablets and creams and injections and things like that which didn't work'*. So, having had lots of tests to reach a diagnosis, Sam felt as if the health professionals were trying out different approaches to managing his pain which was also exhausting and frustrating because they did not work. As Sam developed a deeper understanding of CRPS, he became less scared because he no longer feared that CRPS was life-threatening:

> *So, you know, my mind was saying, 'This is something really, really serious here, you're gonna die from it probably.' I was thinking about strokes and God knows what and I, you know, this is...my...and so yeah, once I got into the pain management team and I just understood more what was going on...it brought my levels down a bit. 'Cos I knew it wasn't killing me. I knew it wasn't... Oh, it is nasty, it is horrible, that sort of thing, but I knew, and that was the biggest thing finding something. I knew. Actually found out what was going on.*

Prior to learning about CRPS, Sam had given it the nickname 'insane pain'. He was angry and upset at finding himself in this inexplicable situation. He was very frustrated at the impact it had had on him. He used humour to show how he coped:

I feel like Dracula sometimes because sunlight can come through the window and the heat from the sunlight (I just keep my feet off). It can set it off. I can feel it radiating out and I'm bursting into flames in my foot.

He said he was unable to walk properly because he had no idea where his left leg was and as a consequence he kept falling over. The CRPS also spread to his hand and he was similarly unable to visualize where his hand was: (*'I was trying to reach for things. I'd miss it by two or three inches'*). Sam described doing *'a lot of visual work'* and as a consequence learned again how to see where his limbs were. He still had to think actively about where his limbs were, but he felt he had markedly improved.

At the time of the interview, he was still more sensitive on his left side. For example, whereas he used to wear his watch on his left wrist, he now wore it on his right. He was also sensitive to wind on his face and the tightness of his footwear, but he felt that the increase in his understanding of his condition had made the pain and burning sensations somehow easier to deal with. In addition, pacing and mindfulness (neither of which he found easy to master) had really helped him to cope well with CRPS. He spent time planning ahead and thinking about his day in order to be in a position to pace himself:

I have to plan it, and I have to work out, you know, how much I've got to do when I get there, how much I can do, how much medication I need to stay. It, it's all, it's all my life [sighs]. I know it sounds sad, but it is centred around CRPS because of the pain.

Sam's life had both shrunk (he was no longer working or doing the things he used to enjoy) and become focused upon managing CRPS. He mentioned motivating himself to do things as a means of distracting himself from the pain, but always underlying everything was the CRPS:

> I have to live with it, I have to work with it. I have to... I have to work with it, rather than work, you know...it is a constant fight against the pain, rather than keep fighting, you work with it, you know.

By 'working with it', Sam said he was referring to planning for different eventualities, whereby he would work around the pain rather than fighting with it:

> I know I'm going to be in pain if I go to the theatre. Theatre seats are very cramped, especially as I'm six foot one, so, it's, it's a bit difficult. So I always say, 'Can I get a seat near the aisle, where I can stick my left leg out?' [laughs] And I'm, you know, I say to myself, 'Look you know what it's going to be like, if you need a break come out of that, if you need to.'

Before he learned these techniques, what he called the 'pain voice' was loud and demanding: 'I'm in pain, I'm in pain. I'm in pain. I can't do that, I'm in pain. I can't do this, I'm in pain.' Applying the mindfulness techniques helped change this focus. Part of this change in outlook came with an increase in confidence, not just in his own ability to cope with CRPS, but also in his ability to cope with other people's attitudes towards his coping behaviour(s). To remain with the theatre example, he had resolved to stand up and move around if he experienced too much pain. He was aware that some people might confront him and question him about his behaviour, and therefore had prepared responses in advance. This preparation made him feel comfortable both with his decision and with his ability to defend himself if challenged.

Sam's interview had a very positive tone to it, but that did not mean that he was not facing a large number of CRPS-related challenges. He spoke of his down days:

> Some mornings you don't get up and not being able to get up, actually physically get out of bed. One, through lack of steam, one through the pain, one through the, you know, you sleep in very strange angles [laughs].

However, for Sam, meeting other people with CRPS was another key turning point. He no longer felt he was battling alone. Sam spoke of the relief he experienced at meeting others with whom he felt he instantly had rapport because they naturally understood what he was going through. He also appreciated being able to reciprocate and in sharing his experiences help them to feel more normal:

> And I could, you know, we could relate to each other and all their stories was the same, the same resonance. So that sort of brought the acceptance all together and then I could deal with it.

It was clear throughout the interview that an important part of Sam's ability to cope was his recognition that no one thing would work all the time; that what was necessary was a range of different coping strategies that he could draw from when he needed:

> Not every part of the medication has helped. Not every part of the physiotherapy helped, and not every part of the pain management has helped. But it has helped with, 10, 20, 30 per cent of it has helped me, which is good, which is great for me. [...] So there's knowledge and there's understanding and there's, err, strategies to deal both with the pain and the thoughts.

Learning to recognize that thoughts were just thoughts was also important. Sam had realized how paralysing negative thinking could be and had learned how to deal with this:

> *Not being horrible, I don't really care what people think about me. I've got no worries about that. 'Cos one of the guys there [on the rehabilitation programme], he was saying he goes on holiday or something with his children, and he got in the swimming pool, and he had a swim and that, 'cos he was having a good day and the next day he was hopping about like a, you know, God knows what, the Hunchback of Notre Dame. And he was really worried about what everybody else around the pool was thinking, you know, and that really upset him. But I don't care. I don't care. If I'm having a good day, I'm gonna enjoy it.*

As a consequence, Sam had developed a straightforward and open way of dealing with other people. He was aware that from the outside he looks healthy and that it is hard to see that there is anything troubling him. If someone asks him, he will simply tell them that he has CRPS, but he has decided that he is not going to worry about what people might be thinking; rather, he will deal with the questions that are directed at him. He chooses to respond in a simple manner: '*I have CRPS, I say that it has damaged my nervous system and I am in pain 24 hours a day.*' Sam actively chooses not to go into detail because '*if you try to explain it in detail, you bore people to death*'. This simple approach enables Sam to manage other people's behaviour and questions, and, in doing so, maintain a level of normality for himself.

SARAH

'It's just not having any answers, why I'm like it now and I never used to be [pause] I think if I had some answers and that...it would stop me thinking about it so much.'

Sarah was 48 years old and had been diagnosed with CRPS in her left leg for two years. At the time of the interview, she worked part-time in a nursing home, lived with her partner and had a close relationship with her grandchild. Three years after the triggering accident, Sarah said she had received a letter which mentioned but did not explain CRPS: *'I was given this label and [...] it wasn't explained, told anything about it or anything. Just had it on a letter and that was it.'* She had had three years of going to 'all these doctors everywhere' and felt that she was not getting answers to any of her questions. The means of conveying the diagnosis was awful, incredibly impersonal and gave her no opportunity to ask questions or to find out more about CRPS. Sarah assumed that the diagnosis was given to her in this way because the doctor himself did not understand CRPS:

> *So I didn't have a clue what it was or anything, nobody explained it, and I think the doctor needs a, I don't think they understand it really. I don't think mine does [laughs].*

Even after diagnosis, Sarah's health professionals had different opinions, which meant they gave conflicting advice (much of it frightening), which in turn had the effect of further confusing Sarah:

> *[...] another doctor said it was vascular disease [laughs] and that I could lose my leg. So that panicked me. So I*

went to see my own doctor and gave her the letter and she put me in touch with Professor XX, so I went to see him, and he said, 'No way is it vascular disease, so it's a damaged nerve, so you need to go on Gabapentin.' So I went back to my doctor and they gave me Gabapentin and it's been quite, not been too bad at the moment.

Sarah felt that she was passed from one health professional to another, each of whom gave conflicting and frightening advice. The lack of 'joined-up' care was really frustrating and extremely time-consuming for Sarah, who seemed to have been both collector and sharer of information as she tried to make sense of the different messages she was being given. She spoke of being given estimates of how long it would take to return to 'normal'. One specialist *'just said, he didn't even look at it [her leg], he just said it will take two years to get better'.* Sarah took him at his word, and although she was not noticing any improvement, she waited for a year and a half. This was a really difficult time for Sarah because she did not feel that it was appropriate to seek further help until the two-year period suggested had passed. Indeed, the sense of abandonment and disempowerment that Sarah felt was really strong through the whole interview. The way in which her diagnosis had been shared with her had coloured her whole experience and she kept coming back to her disappointment that no one had explained anything to her – *'just wrote it on a letter and that was it.'*

Having felt abandoned by the medical profession, Sarah had tried to find out more about CRPS by going on the internet. This was an unhelpful experience because the more she read, the more she began to believe that the pain she experienced was imagined: *'It [the information she found on the internet] had me thinking it was all in my mind.'* The information she found was not helpful and she struggled to explain CRPS to friends and family. She felt that if even her doctors didn't understand it, how could she possibly understand what was happening to her? As a consequence, when she was asked about CRPS, she said that she played it down:

> I don't even say that it is CRPS, I just say my leg's throbbing. I don't really know, I don't know much about it either, not that much, just bits and pieces that I've got on the computer. I don't really understand it, because it is still in my mind. I don't know [laughs resignedly], I don't really know. Nobody has explained it to me or anything. I just read about it, I don't really understand it.

So Sarah lacks the confidence to explain her condition to others, and, on the rare occasions she does say something, she plays it down. The longer Sarah spoke, the clearer it was that she felt completely disempowered. She had a wish for someone to explain CRPS to her, but she lacked the confidence to ask for this to happen. This was after three years of searching for an explanation and traipsing to and from appointments with health professionals. It seemed to Sarah that none of them had checked how much she had understood. She was very confused by the conflicting information and, at the time of the interview, she had begun to doubt that she had CRPS:

> Then another letter saying I had vascular disease [laughs] and that I might lose my leg [laughs], then another one saying it was nerve damage. I still haven't really got an answer now, so it could be a number of things, vascular, nerve damage or CRPS or...

Over time, Sarah became much less mobile. This was problematic for a variety of reasons, not least because she used to go to the gym every day and exercising had been her key means of managing stress. The impact of no longer being able to exercise led to weight gain. Sarah's self-consciousness about her weight gain and her mobility problems led to her isolating herself from her support network: 'All I do is shut myself away in here.' She remembered very clearly going to a specialist and asking them to 'chop the bloody thing off and be done with it'. She had got to the point where she could see no reason to keep her leg; nothing was easing the pain and her leg was fast becoming an encumbrance. For example, she felt that her leg had developed a mind of its own where it 'will walk into things'.

Managing other people's reactions was also difficult. Her family saw that she was looking tired, but didn't understand why. Her partner could not understand why she was no longer so active, and they argued regularly. Sarah was really struggling with the impact of CRPS and had lost her sense of who she was. It took a lot of her energy to go to work, but she also spent a lot of her energy trying to hide just how much CRPS was impacting on her. This acted as a double-edged sword; it enabled her to convince herself that things were normal, but it also served to hide from others close to her just how difficult things were:

> That's it. [...] I used to do a lot of running about for my daughter-in-law and my son. There's a supervisor where I work, he gets ulcerated legs and COPD, so I used to do a lot of running around looking after him. I just think to myself, 'Oh, nobody's doing anything for me.'

The effort of working hard to 'keep it all in' was not something that was sustainable in the longer term and resulted in her feelings seeping out in other ways. Sarah said that she became progressively frustrated that (even though she was hiding her symptoms) her friends and family could not see how much pain she was in. Her frustration was, she thought, the cause of arguments with her partner.

Living with the pain, the isolation, the lack of knowledge about CRPS and the reminders of who she used to be, became increasingly difficult: '*I just can't do anything now, nothing except go to work, and struggle with that. [...] My bike's out in the garage, been there for the last five years.*' Sarah found it more and more difficult to cope and she began to experience the desire to 'just end everything'. She said that she could not cope with the pain anymore, and she felt that there was nowhere for her to turn:

> Just the pain, I couldn't cope with it anymore. Nobody was doing anything [pause], feel like a burden all the time going to the doctors, don't like to keep going to the doctors. Hate it.

At that point, Sarah said she took a combination of pills and alcohol with the intention of ending her life. Her partner found her and called an ambulance and she was taken to hospital. After they got back home, she said that they never spoke about it: '*He don't like talking about things either. He's a very quiet person. I just don't really talk to anyone about it.*' Since then, Sarah said that she has thought about suicide many times, always triggered by the frustration she feels:

> It's just not having any answers, why I'm like it now and I never used to be [pause] I think if I had some answers and that...it would stop me thinking about it so much. Nobody cares is what I think. I think because nobody understands it. But you get to the stage where you think no one bloody understands it.

Sarah continues to do battle with her desire to get more information about CRPS, as well as seeking more understanding from her friends and family. She felt that if she had more information, she would be better able to cope. Her advice to someone else newly diagnosed focused on this: '*Just get lots of information on it, get some answers. Don't just be left like I have without any answers, no information on it.*' When asked how she could go about getting information and answers, however, she became passive: *'I don't know because I haven't. I can't say on that because I don't have any answers. I would love to [laughs].'* She appeared to have given up because of the reaction she received from the health profession – she shows what psychologists would call learned helplessness. In other words, she has been so disempowered by her previous experiences she assumes that there is no point in being proactive:

> *Sarah: People have started noticing it [CRPS] at work.*
>
> *Karen: What do they say?*
>
> *Sarah: They ask me what is wrong with me [laughs].*
>
> *Karen: You are laughing – what do you say?*
>
> *Sarah: I don't tell them about it. I don't even tell them about the CRPS.*
>
> *Karen: So they don't know there is anything wrong with you?*
>
> *Sarah: They do know I have a bad leg, but don't know what is wrong with it. Why have I chosen not to tell them? Because they're going to be the same, I think [...] will probably turn round and say it's all in my head.*

Sarah's story was marked by her sense of helplessness. She had clearly been badly affected by the frustrating process of seeking a clear explanation for her painful leg. This had impacted on her sense of self and her sense of entitlement to information. She seemed to be trapped in a difficult cycle where she tried to hide her CRPS because she had not been understood in the past, and had been accused of the CRPS all being in her mind. However, hiding her CRPS further concealed the hidden condition, which made it harder for her loved ones to appreciate what she was living with. She felt that members of her health team were not aware of her need for further information, but she also said that she did not know how to ask for it and did not want to be a burden to the health team. Sarah's story shows the importance of the person with CRPS and the health team working collaboratively and checking in with one another about the levels of understanding.

MELANIE

*'I think it's just what you need to keep thinking,
that like, if you sit at home and dwell on it, your
pain is still gonna be there. If you go to work, yeah,
your pain is still gonna be there, but at least you
are out meeting people and seeing people.'*

At the time of the interview, Melanie was 22 years old.
She had been diagnosed for two and a half years and
had CRPS in her left leg. She lived with her parents and
worked full-time while also studying towards professional
qualifications. She believed that her CRPS began after she
fell when on holiday. At the time, she thought that she
might have broken her ankle and so went to the Accident
and Emergency department. The X-rays did not identify any
broken bones, and she was given crutches and sent back
to the caravan in which she was holidaying. When she got
home, her foot was no better; she could not bear weight,
was in a lot of pain, which was not relieved by painkillers,
and could not tolerate anything touching her foot. Her
ankle had also twisted into a fixed position. She described
her foot as *'facing inwards. I guess it was, well, I guess a ninety
degree angle'*. She was also realizing that her perception of
her foot was changing:

> *I can remember I think it was really, really swollen and,
> like, my mum and my boyfriend and stuff all said, 'Well, it
> is a little bit, but it isn't that big,' and like I can remember
> my mum saying, like, 'Well I broke my ankle sort of a few
> years ago and it's [Melanie's ankle] nowhere near as
> swollen as that was,' and I was, like, it is huge, so I think*

that from day one, I saw it as like a different image to what everyone else did.

At the time of the interview, Melanie still saw her foot as being different from her non-CRPS foot. She also experienced strong negative feelings towards her foot, and did not feel it was a part of her anymore. Her dislike of her foot was so strong that she would have liked to have had it amputated:

> *You really dislike and don't want it sort of attach...well to you, it's not attached, like you, kind of like, you like, I have sort of disowned it in some way I think. I mean, with the visualization I don't see anything. I have my amputation point and it's these jaggedy lines and that's it, and that's sort of, I find it hard to sort of look at it.*

Melanie's GP diagnosed CRPS about two months after her initial injury. Although this was fast, Melanie felt that he was then unsure about how to proceed: *'He didn't then know what to do with me basically.'* After some investigative tests, Melanie described going online to Google CRPS. It was through this that she found out about the National Centre with expertise in CRPS and asked her GP to refer her.

In the meantime, Melanie was having regular physiotherapy. This is what would usually be prescribed for someone with CRPS; however, the physiotherapists Melanie saw disputed the CRPS diagnosis and treated her as if she did not have CRPS:

> *They didn't agree that I had CRPS, and when I would go to physio they would try to massage it and stuff and it would just be absolute agony. And I'd come away just in sort of agony after physio and that didn't do me any good. So obviously the physio I had before I came into the hospital [for the two-week rehabilitation programme]*

was wasted really because they were saying, 'Oh try and walk on it' and stuff.

This was not helpful because Melanie was struggling to mobilize and was beginning to doubt her diagnosis. She did not feel that the health professionals were listening to her, or hearing what she was telling them. The lack of continuity of care compounded this because Melanie found she had to repeat her story and explain CRPS at each visit:

I find it sounds daft, but I needed to be trained how to walk, not just told that I had to do it because I hadn't obviously, I hadn't done it for a year. So it was very difficult to, to do it really. It was very difficult to do it in the physio that I went to. They weren't very good, and obviously it was a place where you never saw the same one every week, so your session basically spent the first 20 minutes just explaining what was wrong with you, and them saying, 'Oh no, I don't think it's that, it's probably not CRPS, but, erm, I'll just sit here and massage it for 10 minutes [laughs ruefully] and see what happens.' I just used to dig my finger nails onto the bed thing. It was just agony. It was horrible.

Melanie was trying to understand what had happened to her in the face of uncertainty from the health profession. She was having to balance taking enough medication to take the edge off her pain, but ensuring that she did not take too much and compromise her concentration and her ability to continue to work. She was not yet on a permanent contract with her employer and so could not afford to take too much time off work. She was still unable to bear weight *'and just hopped everywhere and didn't really like accept what was going on, I guess'.* She described the wider impact of CRPS as affecting all areas of her life and emphasized the importance of doing things as a means of distracting herself from her pain:

It is difficult, because you kind of like, you don't sleep that great. You're constantly in pain and then having to sort of go to work and do stuff that is, it is hard to sort of keep doing it, but I know that you have to because what is the other option? Just sitting at home? And if, if, I like to keep busy because if I am busy I don't think about the pain as much. Whereas if I'm sat quiet, then obviously the pain's terrible because that's all you can, that's all you've got to think about. Whereas if you try to keep your mind occupied, you sort of, you don't, you obviously know it's still there very bad, but you've got something to keep your mind busy without having to accept the pain.

Keeping busy was one of Melanie's key coping strategies; however, this became harder once she was no longer able to drive. She felt that she was gradually losing more and more of her independence. This was very hard because, at only 22 years old, she was just beginning to carve out her own life and build her independence: '*If you want something and you are used to doing it when you want it, it's hard to wait however long it takes, for the person you've asked to then do it.*' Having to ask someone else to do something for her that pre-CRPS she would have done without thinking was hard enough. Waiting for them to do this thing in their own time was harder. So, not only do you have to get used to asking for help, you also need to be prepared for the fact that help might not be delivered as fast as you would like:

It's just silly things, like if you want something, like something passed to you or something. You want it then, but it's difficult because obviously if they are doing something then you've got to wait for them and it's, so it's like it is hard to be patient with as well, because obviously if it wasn't for the condition you would be able, you wouldn't have to rely on other people for everything.

She also found it much harder to be spontaneous:

Socially it is very hard because you have to, you have to plan everywhere you go. You can't just turn up somewhere without knowing what the place is like. You need to know sort of, like if there's lifts? Is there lots of seating?

Melanie had found a few restaurants that she felt comfortable in, and would only accept invitations that involved these places. At the time of the interview, the thought of going to a new place was too much because there would be too many unknowns. Would there be a long wait? If so, would there be somewhere she could sit? How busy would it be? Would there be steps? Just thinking about these things made Melanie anxious and she had noticed that increased anxiety went hand in hand with an increase in her pain. She had noticed that this was beginning to have an impact on her life, which she felt was shrinking as she lost her independence and her confidence in her ability to deal with new situations and places. She had also noticed that she was engaging in 'what-iffing' (imagining possible scenarios and worrying about them). This in itself was also exhausting: *'It makes you quite tired, and obviously 'cos your pain is higher, you're getting more tired.'*

Melanie talked about how difficult she found it to pace her activities. Her attitude was to try to 'get on with things', but this could have negative consequences, in that her pain levels increased so much that she needed to rest for a couple of days. She was constantly monitoring and evaluating how much energy she had to 'spend':

So I had a really good night on the Saturday, but then the consequence was two days pretty much with my foot up because I was in so much pain all the time, I really couldn't do anything. It's just Catch-22 really, because anything you sort of so, you get consequences for it basically.

This need to pace clashed with her desire to try to maintain some normality in her life. She was quite clear that she understood there was no magic cure and that, as a consequence, she had two choices: one to try to get on with her life, and the other to sit and wait and hope for a cure:

> I'm young, I'm only 22. I don't want to, there's no cure for this at the moment. I'm quite logical and quite realistic, and like at the moment there isn't a cure and I don't want to be sort of sat at home and waiting for a cure that might or might not come along, and then ruin the rest of my life.

So, although pacing was not something she felt she managed well, she consciously took this approach knowing that lack of pacing meant she experienced what she called 'payback'. She focused on her work and tried to fit in her social life, her family and her study too. She spoke of occasionally 'crashing', but felt that her system worked for her:

> I know it's not necessarily the right way to do it, but it seems to work for me. [...] I still manage to get most things I need to done. So I don't sort of, I mean I still see friends, see family, sort of make time for people and still work and still study, so it does sort of, I think it works.

Melanie also sought alternative means of coping, and found that acupuncture worked well for her because it helped with relaxation and reduced her pain. She also discovered that sun beds were helpful: she found the heat eased her pain. She was aware of the potential risks of using sun beds regularly, but felt that the benefits outweighed the potential costs. Working towards acceptance of her CRPS was a process that she could see she was in, but could not see how she could achieve. She was very aware of the difference between knowledge and acceptance. It was one thing to know something, but a very different experience to accept it:

You've obviously been told everything what's going on and stuff, but to sort of get on with life you kind of have to just ignore it in some aspects and get on with it. Then you don't wanna do that, you wanna accept that this is happening...it is just everything like Catch-22 with everything you do with it.

Life had very much become a juggling act. Trying to balance all the competing demands of a normal busy life when CRPS is introduced into the equation is not easy. Incorporating therapy in her busy life was done on a 'see-saw' basis:

It's sort of like, when you are not working you can do your therapy and kind of like it [CRPS] may improve quicker, but when you're at work your therapy suffers a little bit because obviously you're at work the majority of the day and it's hard to... When you come home the therapy that you are doing probably isn't as good quality because you are knackered from work basically.

In spite of all this, Melanie worked hard at maintaining a positive attitude as well as her social contacts:

I think it's just what you need to keep thinking, that like, if you sit at home and dwell on it, your pain is still gonna be there. If you go to work, yeah, your pain is still gonna be there, but at least you are out meeting people and seeing people.

THOMAS

*'I didn't know anything – the help I needed. If I needed
any help. If what I was doing was right. Because
there was research on the internet that said it was
right, and there was research that said it wasn't.'*

Thomas was 30 years old at the time of the interview.
He had been diagnosed for two years. CRPS was in his
right leg as well as both arms. He lived with his wife and
two-year-old daughter. Thomas described being in a state
of fear and uncertainty as he searched for an explanation
for his symptoms:

> *I didn't know what I was dealing with and then you just
> tend to go on the internet and it gives you all those
> things, information, and it's a bit overwhelming really.*

His assumption was that his symptoms would clear up
by themselves; indeed, this was consistent with the
information he had found online. However, his symptoms
did not disappear after six months – a cut-off point he had
read about on the internet:

> *What it says is that it tends to go away within six months,
> and if it doesn't go away, you're stuck with it [CRPS]
> for life. And then it is all doom and gloom after the six
> months.*

So Thomas veered from optimism to despair as time passed.
The despair was worsened by the lack of CRPS-related
knowledge displayed by the health professionals with
whom Thomas interacted. No one could explain clearly to
Thomas what CRPS was. This led to him experiencing a

high level of anxiety about the correct way to manage his symptoms. He spoke about receiving conflicting messages from healthcare professionals and from the different sites he looked at online:

> I didn't know anything – the help I needed. If I needed any help. If what I was doing was right. Because there was research on the internet that said it was right, and there was research that said it wasn't.

Thomas was left in the difficult position of navigating his way through the conflicting advice and information, whilst trying at the same time to judge the quality of the information he was finding. He felt very alone. He said it felt as if no one understood and no one could help. He was really frustrated about the length of time it took to reach a diagnosis because much of the information online emphasized the need for a speedy diagnosis in order to maximize the chance of recovering.

However, even with a diagnosis, there were conflicting approaches. Many of the health professionals he saw wanted to treat his pain with medication. Thomas had concerns about this; he had learned from experience that, at best, medication took the edge off his pain, and, more often than not, the side effects left him drowsy. This was a problem for a number of reasons, not least because he was looking after his two-year-old daughter while his wife worked. He could not afford to be drowsy because this could put her safety at risk. He felt that this need was not heard by the doctors treating him and he felt pressured to follow this advice whilst feeling that his opinion did not count:

> They said if you are not having the injection in your spine, you don't want Tramadol and whatever else, then there is nothing we can do for you. So I decided to go ahead with the injection in my spine.

As a consequence, Thomas felt as if the medical professional had abandoned him. He felt that the doctors believed it was his fault that the medication did not work, and that this was why he was jettisoned by the system: *'I just felt that it was like a quick fix and if it doesn't work, you are on your own.'* He also felt that the health professionals he was seeing did not take his life as a whole into account but just focused on the symptom of pain. As mentioned before, he had learned through experience that if he took Tramadol regularly he would be *'zonked out: that's what Tramadol does to me; I'm there, but I'm not there'.*

He felt that the health professionals thought he was being difficult because he did not want to take the medicine. He said that one doctor commented: *'If you do not take painkillers, it is because you want to feel pain isn't it?'* Thomas was exasperated that the health professional could not understand the logic behind his decision not to take Tramadol: *'If I'm in this much pain and I'm not taking painkillers, there's a good reason behind it.'* So Thomas and his doctor were at an impasse. The doctor was frustrated because Thomas was questioning and resisting his recommendation, whereas Thomas was feeling disempowered because he was not being listened to, heard or understood.

Other health professionals had clearly felt disempowered themselves because there was so little that they could do to help. For example, Thomas said that his GP had apologized for not being able to help and expressed the wish that he could help make Thomas better. This was actually really difficult for Thomas to hear and, in fact, had the effect of making him feel guilty for being a patient who (a) could not be fixed and (b) challenged the GP's image of himself as a healer.

In terms of treatment, Thomas's mother-in-law had found reference to the Mineral Hospital as being a place of national expertise with respect to CRPS. This was exciting news because help was now tangible. However, optimism and excitement were dashed when Thomas presented his GP with the information and discovered that the GP was already aware of the existence of the hospital. The fact that the GP had apologized for not being able to help but had not referred Thomas to a place with expertise in treating his condition was galling. However, Thomas did not feel that he could confront his GP about this for fear of ruining what he considered was a good relationship. This highlights the huge power differential: since the GP is a gatekeeper who can facilitate access to help, Thomas did not feel able to express his true feelings:

> Why wasn't I referred earlier? I never asked this. I thought I've got a good relationship with him and I don't want to ruin it, because he will probably just make me really angry.

Finally attending a CRPS rehabilitation programme and meeting health professionals who understood *and* worked regularly with people who had CRPS was a relief. Getting access to information about CRPS helped Thomas to make sense of his own CRPS-related experiences, and consequently his confidence at being able to explain CRPS to others grew. Access to resources, such as a bookmark developed by the (now closed) CRPS@themin group was especially useful (the bookmark clearly explained what CRPS is and how best to help someone who has CRPS):

> And the thing is, it went from not being able to explain it to my closer friends who used to know me for what I was: from working 60–70 hours a week and being a proper workaholic, to not being able to make a cup of tea. And it helped explain it, it really did. I just gave them a card [bookmark] and all of a sudden, I've got my friends going 'Fucking hell, I didn't realize it was that bad.'

The downside of becoming more informed was that this encouraged friends and family to ask more questions. Questions could be overwhelming, not least because the focus was on CRPS rather than on Thomas, and the temptation was to say, 'Go on the bloody internet and look it up.' Handling questions from others could be exhausting, and whilst Thomas recognized that the questions reflected concern on the part of the questioner, fielding these questions was tiring. In addition, the unpredictability of CRPS in conjunction with the unremitting pain was an aspect that Thomas found especially hard to cope with:

> You never know, you never know, you don't know if you are going to be able to get out of bed. If you do get out of bed OK (whatever OK is), you come downstairs, you have your cup of tea and you don't know if you are going to be able to get up and do something.

Thomas described CRPS as striking at his identity and his masculinity because he was no longer working. His role in the family had changed beyond recognition, and he no longer knew who he was. He especially struggled with what he called 'reminders' that he faced each day:

> There are those reminders like when you start trying to get up to do this or get up to do that and you feel the reminders – you feel the reminder – hold on a minute – I'm not that person – you can't just go on and do it.

Thomas began to contemplate taking his own life. He felt that this had become the only option available to him. He could see the impact his condition was having on his family and he thought that if he removed himself from the picture they would have a chance of 'being normal'. Thomas took pills – 'however many I could get my hands on at the time'. He was rushed to hospital. Treated, assessed by the crisis team and discharged. The crisis team arranged for follow-up family therapy, which Thomas said he had found helpful. In particular, the therapy helped Thomas to talk more openly with his partner about how he was feeling. He still finds himself fighting the suicidal thoughts, but the motivation has changed from a desire to end his life to a desire to escape the pain for a short time:

> *I never thought it would be possible to live with this amount of pain. Erm, that's it, really it. There are days when you think, for fuck's sake, give me a break.*

Thomas's story is very much like a rollercoaster; adapting to living with CRPS involved lurching from hope and optimism to the depths of despair as he navigated the uncertain world he found himself in. Thomas's interactions with health professionals were disempowering; for example, learning that health professionals don't have all the answers and don't know how to help can be a shock. Finding out that health professionals offer conflicting advice or don't seem to see you as a whole person is disorientating. Many health professionals whom Thomas encountered tried to focus on reducing the pain, but neglected to see the negative impact the side effects of their treatment was having on Thomas's wider life. Key to his progress was finding health professionals who listened and heard his story, believed his explanation of his symptoms and were honest about their ability to help.

CRYSTAL

'Sex. Sex is the answer. But you can't keep doing it,
because there is things to be done during the day!'

Crystal was 44 years old at the time of the interview. She had been diagnosed for two years. CRPS was in her right arm, both shoulders and in her left leg. She lived with her partner. Crystal injured her right arm in a car accident and said that the pain simply would not go away. She said that it took about a year from accident to diagnosis; this year was marked by numerous medical appointments which she found both time-consuming and emotionally exhausting. The range of appointments and exploratory tests actually identified a number of other health conditions which in themselves were frightening:

> ...and they found other things wrong with me, erm, abnormal blood cells. I had lymph glands come up. I had lumps removed because they thought it was lymphoma, so I had lumps taken out of the neck and the groin. So, as they are investigating the arm, they found, they opened a big bag of other things that came out.

Naturally, this led to Crystal experiencing high levels of anxiety about her health, exacerbated by the constant pain she was living with, which was still unexplained and worsening:

> The pain was getting worse, and the circulation was getting worse, and the hand was getting colder. It was changing colour, erm, the skin was going funny, skin was cracking. All different things were happening to me.

It was not surprising that Crystal began to feel that she was losing control. She was regularly attending medical appointments, and all the time her symptoms were worsening. At the same time, the tests were not producing any answers and Crystal began to doubt herself. Were the symptoms all in her mind? The sense that she was losing control led Crystal to pay closer attention to her symptoms and she monitored her body all the time. Every time she noticed a new pain or a change, it became a sign that something terrible was happening:

> *I got it in my head that I was having a stroke, and I kept saying to them; I kept thinking my mouth is dropping. Do you know what I mean? So, I like, I would go around 'my mouth is dropping, my mouth is dropping'.*

Eventually, Crystal was diagnosed with CRPS, but this was not as helpful as she had hoped; she found it hard to understand what CRPS was, and she was still worried that she might have something life-threatening such as bone cancer. The year of toing and froing between appointments had made her doubt her sanity:

> *I really thought I was going mad and I thought I was making it up.*

Dealing with all the health professionals was exhausting, and because Crystal had all but convinced herself that she was 'mad' or somehow 'making it up', she stopped asking health professionals to explain what they were saying. This meant that she only picked up little bits of the whole picture because she did not double-check her understanding. Only picking up on little bits of the story increased Crystal's anxiety and fed her fear about the worst-case scenarios that she was imagining:

I just sit there and do 'Yeah, yeah, yeah. Oh yeah, yeah' and then go out and then [partner's name] will go, 'What did they say?' and I haven't got a clue what's been said, to be honest. I don't actually know, but they did say something about the blood cells.

In terms of managing her pain, Crystal self-medicated, preferring to take medication when she felt she needed it, rather than by following a timetable. She had in effect become an expert at managing her drugs. This worked for her when she was at home, but proved problematic on the occasions when she was admitted to hospital. Her approach clashed with the hospital's approach:

...because I was in pain at night, and I would ask for my medication and they said, 'No, you have had it at a certain time, can you hang on for another...' Well no! I want it now because I'm going to get worse in about half an hour. It is going to get worse, I know what's going to happen. But they wouldn't issue it to me.

This experience confirmed Crystal's sense of lack of control and made her feel as if her expertise and experience of dealing with her condition counted for nothing. The mismatch between her ability to manage her pain at home versus the sense of her control being taken away whilst in hospital was hard to cope with, leading to frustration, which in turn raised her pain levels. Crystal was very aware that she had not been following protocol, but at the same time she felt that the health professionals in hospital had not understood the impact of CRPS:

I suppose they were doing it the right way. I do it the wrong way. I know I do it the wrong way. I just bang them [tablets] down my neck like sweets now. They were doing it the right way, but I felt like they looked at me, nobody, I don't think nobody knows enough about CRPS.

So the lack of knowledge about CRPS amongst health professionals also led to Crystal feeling disempowered. This explains her tendency to pretend that she understands, rather than ask questions of health professionals. She described switching off when she talked about her encounters with the less well-informed members of the health profession. It was too tiring for her to have to explain that she had CRPS and then to explain how it manifests: '*I can't be bothered to explain now, can't be bothered because they* should *know.*' This highlights the chasm between what Crystal felt health professionals should know and her experience of how little they appeared to know about CRPS.

In addition, Crystal found trying to explain CRPS to others exhausting. In particular, meeting new people was especially stressful because she was uncertain about how they might react. As such, she engaged in a lot of 'what-iffing':

> *Say if one day we're out somewhere and then halfway through I say that I don't feel very well? I don't want to ruin it for them. And say we have got to turn round and go back, or I don't want them to see me doubled up in pain because people don't know how to handle it?*

So Crystal can be paralysed by fear that her friends will be embarrassed and not understand what is happening, or that her CRPS will impose on her friends' experience too. She herself was unsure about how to proceed; she feared that explaining her experiences to others would make her come across as 'attention seeking'. She was very concerned with how others might perceive her, and this fear led her to behave in ways that were not helpful for the management of her pain. For example, rather than tell friends that she had had enough and wanted to return home, she will force herself to stay out:

I will sit there and watch them go through, get all this happiness and that, and I'm sitting there cringing and really wanting to go, and forcing back the tears.

In neglecting her own needs, she gets increasingly stressed, which in turn increases the pain she experiences and makes the situation much harder to deal with. Crystal had great insight into what was happening, but her desire to avoid impacting on others made her react in ways that hid how she was really feeling. Indeed, hiding was another strategy she used to cope, but the problem with isolating herself was that this allowed her negative thoughts to spiral and to grow. During our interview, Crystal reflected on this strategy and recognized that one of the dangers of not talking to others about her feelings was that her mind could 'play tricks':

Like now when I talk it through with you level-headedly, I think 'Crystal, you bloody idiot! You have got so much going on.' Do you know what I mean? It's like the devil on your shoulder.

How she feels about herself and how she fears she impacts on others, along with the intensity of the CRPS pain and the despair of not knowing when it will end, led to her considering suicide as an option. Crystal found that she was able to cope with her pain for a certain length of time, but if the intensity and duration increased, *'something clicks in your head and you think "No! I've had it now. That's it."'* She described these moments as coming upon her without warning – the 'click' in her head was impulsive. This impulsivity scared her:

I sort of frighten myself sometimes, 'cos I'm like, oh my God, say if I do overstep the mark and suddenly decided in a fleeting moment just like that, you know?

She had developed a number of strategies to help ride these impulsive and compulsive feelings. One was to ensure that she had photographs of her loved ones around her to remind herself of how much they care for her, and she for them. She also found that self-harm helped her to feel as if she was taking back some control:

> That's when self-harm comes in, 'cos it is me controlling it then. It's me controlling me. I'm putting in the pain [...] instead of whatever's happening to me inside not taking over. I'm not alienated, being alienated by whatever it is. I'm controlling it.

Crystal therefore felt more able to control the pain that *she* inflicted, which served to distract her from the CRPS pain. She visualized the CRPS pain as an alien that had taken over the inner workings of her body and saw self-harm as a means of directly attacking her CRPS – the self-harm was directed towards the area where her CRPS pain was worse: 'the arm'. She used the term 'the' rather than 'my' because her arm no longer felt as if it was a part of her:

> If the pain is bad on the arm, then I will attack the arm. I've put cigarettes out on my arm. I've cut it, erm, I've made plans for how to amputate the arm.

Crystal no longer recognized her arm as belonging to her when she looked at it. This was disconcerting to say the least; she can see her arm, but she does not see 'it' as belonging to her:

> When I look at the arm, to me it still doesn't look like my arm. If I put the arm here like that [out of her line of sight], I can't feel that the arm is there.

She mentioned that meeting other people with CRPS had been helpful, but also pointed out that this could be a mixed blessing; finding others with similar experiences helped her to feel more normal, but could also be negative:

> There are people with CRPS and they walk around with these walking frames which frightens the life out of me. I ain't doing that. There was a bloke that has his leg up and he hadn't felt his leg for years and it was blue and he hadn't walked for I don't know how long. And then I thought, 'Oh my God. I can't do that.'

So, seeing others who have CRPS but who struggle with mobility was frightening because it led to Crystal worrying that this also might be in store for her:

> 'Cos I stare at them and think please don't let me be like that. Please don't let me be like that. Do you know what I mean? It frightens me.

Finally, one strategy that had a really positive impact on the CRPS pain, which Crystal shared towards the end of our interview, was that sex was a really good coping strategy. She explained that orgasm completely blocks the pain. She was rueful that sex was not a practical cure:

> Sex. Sex is the answer. But you can't keep doing it, because there is things to be done during the day!

STELLA

'So, I treated it almost like a project. She [the
physiotherapist] said four times a day so four times a
day, whatever I was doing, I would stop and do these
exercises. And my eyes would be streaming because it
was so painful. But it worked, you know. It worked.'

Stella was 65 years old and had been diagnosed for three
years at the time of the interview. She had had CRPS in her
left arm, but felt that her CRPS had largely resolved. Her
CRPS had started when she broke her elbow and was put
into a plaster cast from her shoulder down to her fingers:

> I had this terrible panic because I could feel my arm was
> swelling and I, I think that might have been the start of
> it. And it was like my arm was swelling. That's a nuisance,
> it's [the cast], it has got to come off now. And it felt
> claustrophobic, I have terrible claustrophobia and it felt
> like my arm was getting claustrophobia. And I literally
> had to go to A&E and the time I was waiting, in my head
> I was panicking so much. And whether that was the start
> of it, erm, I don't know.

Stella also had what she described as 'blue sausage, huge
blue fingers' and although she talked to the nurses in A&E
about this, she said that they had no idea what was causing
the problem other than assuming it was linked directly
to her broken elbow. She described having a number
of follow-up appointments. At the third appointment a
potential diagnosis was offered, but the way in which the
information was delivered was incredibly insensitive and
unhelpful:

And then on the third appointment the doctor said (I was furious with them afterwards), 'Watch those fingers it might be...' and then he rattled off a phrase that didn't mean a thing to me and said, 'You need physio for that,' and that was all that was said.

Later in the interview, she said that she had returned to the original doctor and had tried to tell him that she wished he had explained CRPS more clearly to her when he had first mentioned it as a possibility:

I said, 'You said, you know 'cos I've now found out why I've got these blue fingers and you should have explained it to me,' erm, and he looked at his notes and said, 'Look, I've written I've given a full and thorough explanation of CRPS to this patient' or something. I said, 'You didn't say ten words, watch those fingers, you might have Complex Regional Pain Syndrome,' and I said that wasn't good enough. I was so upset I was in floods of tears. He did apologize, but if he'd just said, 'Oh, I've just noticed your fingers' [...] erm, I think that would have cut through all the nonsense I went through afterwards trying to find out about it.

This highlights the importance of health professionals checking their patients' understanding of the information they have been given. The health professional who had diagnosed Stella thought he had explained CRPS clearly to her and was surprised when she challenged him at a later date. It is important to remember that patients are often feeling anxious and may not remember all that they have been told.

Stella felt that she had been left to organize her own physiotherapy. She discovered that there was a waiting list of three months for NHS physiotherapy treatment and so she decided to turn to the private sector. The person she spoke to said that she could be seen in an hour and a half from when she made her phone call. At this appointment, CRPS was explained fully to Stella: *'She [the private physiotherapist] said, "Oh, we've got some work to do there" and then explained what it was.'* After this initial session, Stella said that she turned to the internet and *'frightened the life out of myself.* This was a really disturbing experience and she came away in a state of extreme anxiety and was afraid that she could lose her arm: *'Oh God! All sorts of scenarios were going through my head.'* However, her private physiotherapist explained that Stella needed to learn to work through the pain and to complete the exercises prescribed. Stella decided to take a proactive approach to her rehabilitation:

> *So I treated it almost like a project. She [the physiotherapist] said four times a day so, four times a day, whatever I was doing, I would stop and do these exercises. And my eyes would be streaming because it was so painful. But it worked, you know. It worked.*

She would do the recommended exercises wherever she was. Stella recounted being at a friend's house, and at the allotted time for her exercises, she asked her friend if she could make use of the spare room for a few minutes:

> *I thought if I don't do what I am told on this, I'm going to pay the consequences. I didn't know what the consequences would be, but, I just think I had faith in this physio, she was so good, you know and, erm, she was very reassuring and, erm, I do think she, in fact the fact is she got me through it. Which sounds a bit dramatic, doesn't it? But I think there's a reality there.*

Stella said that gradually over a few months she noticed improvement. At the time of the interview, three years on from the initial onset of CRPS, she said that her pain was much much lower and that the key symptoms she had were a 'fizzing', which felt as though her arm had been plunged into a 'load of nettles', and itching that she found very difficult to stop herself from scratching. She said that she experienced this up to eight times a day. Initially, Stella had closely monitored the fizzing symptoms, to the extent that she would time how long each episode lasted. However, she decided that this was not a helpful strategy and was in fact leading her to focus more on the symptoms:

> It was working out at about every 2 hours [...] and I just thought life is too short to time everything [laughs]. It was probably six or eight times a day [...] not that long, 10 minutes.

Stella had also noticed that her affected hand smelled differently:

> Has anybody ever said that their arm smells different when it's got CRPS? Which is a weird thing to say, I know. I can smell my hand, I mean now. I didn't even realize your skin smelt; I have a shower every day [laughs], erm, and, erm, my hands smelt differently when I had CRPS.

She had also noticed a drastic change in how she perceived her arm. 'I said to my husband "My arm feels like a flipper, it doesn't feel like an arm."' She grew to really dislike her arm to the extent that a few months after she had broken her elbow:

> I couldn't bear this thing on me anymore. I, it had, I had to get away from it. [...] I had this thing on me and this is so strange and hard to understand, [...] and erm, I had to get away from this thing that was attached to me, erm, and I couldn't.

She tried to reason with herself about her situation, telling herself to calm down and reminding herself that, regardless of how she felt, it was the same arm she had always had. She spoke with her physiotherapist, who suggested Stella try mirror therapy and to focus on actively liking her hand: '*I had to love my hand. I spent hours telling, and my arm, stroking it and telling it what a lovely arm it was [laughs].*' Stella said that it took about seven months to feel more 'normal' about her arm and hand. She reflected on the problems she had experienced before her CRPS had resolved. She spoke about the all-encompassing nature of the pain and the frustration of not being able to do things 'properly'. She described her hand as having a mind of its own:

> *I remember picking up a mug once, I was working, I was back at work, erm, although I didn't really take much time off, erm, and, erm, I was making a cup of tea for the managing director and I dropped it [her voice became quite emotional here] because I used both hands, erm, and I dropped the mug and it went everywhere and I thought (I did it the other day), this hand seems to have a mind of its own.*

She was frustrated about all the things she was no longer able to do: she used to have a business, but could no longer run it; she could not knit or play the piano because her ability to do tasks that needed fine finger movements was lost. In spite of this, she was determined to work through the pain. Her physiotherapist had told her that:

> *There was no cause for the pain, this is how she explained it if I remember it correctly, there was no cause for the pain, it was almost as if your brain hadn't switched off the pain signal. So there was nothing causing the pain, so therefore you had to ignore it, and [she said] these exercises would restore function.*

Although this information was counterintuitive, it was also liberating, and Stella felt that she had permission to push herself through the pain. She learned strategies to keep her hand flexible; for example, she discovered that going to bed with her hand open and resting on her thigh stopped her hand from closing in the night. If she neglected to do this, she had terrible trouble opening her fingers in the morning. So, through advice and experimentation, Stella found ways to cope. She took up knitting again using larger needles and kept a detailed diary throughout her CRPS journey. The diary allowed her to vent her negative feelings. She also tried to direct her 'no-nonsense' attitude towards her situation: '*I was determined that I'd got to sort this. I hadn't got time to faff around you know. It had to be sorted.*' This was not easy and Stella recognized how difficult it was to stay positive. She said she was concerned about how others might be feeling and reacting and so did not want to worry them, or become a burden to them:

> *And people don't want you being always miserable in front of them. My husband had enough to cope with me having it, let alone being a bit sort of down, you know, certainly not depressed, but a bit...when you are in pain and your life is a bit restricted, you are not going to go around with a great beaming smile, are you?*'

She said that she had felt very down about three or four weeks after her CRPS symptoms began, but she applied the same proactive coping strategy to this experience:

> *I just thought, hang on, I'm not going to go along that road. You know, I just know this is something, and, erm, then I would have a strategy to find something to do. I'm pretty busy anyway so that wasn't difficult. But if I was just sort of moping I think, 'OK, you can't go along that road, you don't want to add depression to the mix, you know, do you?' So I just sort it. I think maybe if you were*

not so strong, if you were a bit depressed anyway, you wouldn't have that mental strength to keep yourself up.

For Stella, three years on from her diagnosis, she considered the CRPS to have almost gone. She put this down to her determination to do the exercises recommended (even when they hurt), to having the finances to access private physiotherapy, and, in so doing, to getting faster treatment than was available via the NHS. She also recognized the difficulty but emphasized the importance of keeping positive.

SNOOPY

'I suppose a lot of people would have, erm, given up, and rolled over, and just let their house, their personal everything be unkempt and just given up on the world. And I think "No!" I am a battler, a survivor really. I don't want to be a victim. That is one thing I don't want to be, a victim.'

Snoopy was 46 years old at the time of the interview. She had been diagnosed for just over a year. She had CRPS in both her legs. She lived alone. Following an accident at work that resulted in her twisting her ankle, she had physiotherapy, but her pain continued to worsen. She was given MRI scans and was operated on a year and a half after her initial injury. After the operation, she had to wear a plaster cast for about 14 weeks. Tolerating the cast was really difficult because of the pain she was experiencing and she had the cast removed and a new one fitted three times. When the cast was finally removed, she was offered further physiotherapy, but her pain was too great and she began to experience other symptoms, including blood blisters and her foot swelling up. She returned to her surgeon who suggested that she might have CRPS, and although his surgical job was complete, he asked her to keep in touch because he was interested in learning more about CRPS:

'Cos even though he's surgically fixed my ankle, he still wants to keep me on his books because he's interested in my journey with the, with the CRPS.

Snoopy was grateful for what she described as a fast diagnosis and quick referral to Bath, but found that her employers lacked both understanding and empathy:

> The [work] doctor's been an absolute nightmare. He doesn't, well, he doesn't believe I've even had the surgery, but that is a separate story. But that has been quite, erm. The journey, with, you know, the problems with him not accepting that has been most problematic. But all the NHS people have been fantastic really.

Snoopy discovered that her employer had 'had me under medical surveillance for a number of months, well obviously he must have had doubts about my condition'. Battling with this lack of understanding and disbelief was tiring, to say the least. She coped by reminding herself of the validity of her symptoms:

> Well, I think to myself, because I know it is 100 per cent genuine. I've got, you know, all the medical evidence. I've got heat scans and, you know, I've had so many different doctors.

Her employer's response was not just undermining; it was also extremely disappointing. Snoopy was sad that after her many years of service they would react in this way at a time when she needed support and understanding: 'It saddens me that that's the route they've taken, after you know, 24 years' service'. As a consequence, at the time of the interview, Snoopy was in the process of medically retiring from her job.

An issue she said she found especially difficult was that of maintaining her independence. Up until the CRPS, Snoopy had been independent and very active. Prior to CRPS, friends would ask how she was and what she had been up to and she would reel off a long list of activities. '[...] and they would say "You make me tired just thinking, just *listening to what you have been [doing]".* So CRPS had been life-changing. She was retiring from her job and was no longer able to engage spontaneously in activities (both pleasurable as well as chores that she used to do). This led to high levels of frustration: at not being able to do things, at having to ask other people to do things (or to pay for jobs to be done that previously she would have done herself), and because other people did not do things to the high standard Snoopy expected. Frustration went hand in hand with loss:

> *It's like my two little dogs. They go out with the dog walker. She's lovely, I've known her for years. She picks them up and they are happy as Larry. They just went off as I came down here. But the enjoyment of putting my two dogs on the lead and taking them out myself has gone.*

Snoopy spoke of having been house bound for seven months, when she had been unable to drive her manual vehicle. She had eventually decided to invest in a mobility scooter, which had begun to make a difference. Having been unable to go far from her house, she was now able to go to the local supermarket which was two miles away. Snoopy's life began to expand again, and she started to think about the challenges she faced and how she could address them:

> *I thought long-term, if I am not getting any better, that's when I thought, well, I'm gonna have to sell my car and get an automatic. Then having an automatic car I could drive to the supermarket, but then I need my scooter to get round the store or like to go to the garden centre. You can drive there, but there's getting round inside and you know, I think, socially I don't go out an awful lot because it's very hard work.*

Initially it was hard to come to terms with being a person who needed a mobility scooter – in Snoopy's mind, they were for elderly people. She coped by choosing a black scooter that she could accessorize with her favourite colours. She said that it took a while for her to realize that nobody else took much notice of the fact that she was on a scooter. She became aware that worrying about what people *might* be thinking meant she was using energy that could be focused elsewhere. Although she felt very self-conscious at first, once she recognized that others were not noticing, her confidence grew:

> *The first time I went out on it I felt really quite self-conscious and embarrassed really. I mean now I can go in my little corner-shop and they don't take any notice and I whizz round and I can queue up. I can go right up to the Post Office counter and do things. But, yeah. It is quite embarrassing going up to. I even feel quite embarrassed sometimes getting my big bags of medication from the chemist, 'cos I've never been a person that took tablets.*

So it took great effort and courage to actually leave the house and then to get around at the destination. Snoopy found dealing with CRPS overwhelming at first and drew from coping strategies she had learned prior to CRPS. Snoopy's mother used to tell her, 'Don't think about how far you've got to go, think about how far you have come.' Snoopy has tried to maintain a positive outlook throughout her CRPS journey:

> *I suppose a lot of people would have, erm, given up, and rolled over, and just let their house, their personal everything be unkempt and just given up on the world. And I think 'No!' I am a battler, a survivor really. I don't want to be a victim. That is one thing I don't want to be, a victim.*

For Snoopy, being a victim would be someone who sat at home and did nothing – someone who allowed the condition to totally overwhelm them. She said that at times CRPS did overwhelm her, particularly when 'my legs are burning and, you know, I've had burning right up my legs, my whole body felt like it's being cremated alive'. Her focus, however, was very much on learning to live with CRPS: *'However much I don't want to have CRPS, I've got it and the fact is just learning the best you can to, erm, live with it.'* This involved the concept of acceptance, something which she spoke of continuing to work towards. Her sheer determination to cope was both positive and negative, because whilst determination can motivate you to carry on, it can sometimes interfere with an ability to pace. Snoopy referred to an activity analysis she had completed whilst on the CRPS rehabilitation programme. This had highlighted periods of high-intensity activity which Snoopy found difficult to change:

> *It's alright saying 'pace yourself', but there's certain things that you have to do, erm. And being a very busy, active person, that is what I find the hardest.*

And although she was aware of the negative impact of not pacing, prioritizing relaxation was not easy. However, this awareness led her to think more creatively about how to cope, as well as how to adapt to life with CRPS:

> *But, erm, I've got to try to adapt and think well. This is who I am as well, and my life's just different now. It is no good sitting there and thinking 'I used to get up there and do all that wallpapering' or this, that and the other. I'm not doing that so I'll have to work about the coping strategies.*

WHAT CAN WE LEARN FROM THESE PEOPLE'S STORIES?

What I hope these stories show is that everyone experiences CRPS in their own unique way; just because one person has one set of symptoms, it does not mean that you will have these symptoms too. Your CRPS is your own journey. However, you will also have noticed that there are many similarities across the stories, and I hope that reading these people's stories, experiences and journeys will, in a way, be reassuring because you may well find out that you are not alone in your personal CRPS experiences.

You will have read that many have spoken about the difficult time they had from the onset of their symptoms, as they were bounced from health professional to health professional, each professional trying to work out what it was that was causing the problem. These ten people spoke of feeling that they were imagining their symptoms, and all spoke of relief on diagnosis at finding out that they were not going mad. All found it difficult to live with CRPS; it is not life-threatening, but it is life-changing, and they shared a variety of coping strategies that they had tried out.

Indeed, dealing with all the challenges that come with CRPS can be a very testing time which can lead to high levels of frustration and anger. Finding ways to cope with these powerful emotions is important. Indeed, the whole process of coping with CRPS is emotionally demanding and can impact on an individual's self-esteem, sense of well-being and ability to concentrate and remember things. Many also experience periods of depression and fear for the future, and some become so low that they experience suicidal thoughts. Psychological support is therefore really important. The next chapter of this book explores psychology-based coping strategies that people living with CRPS have found helpful.

Chapter 3

HOW CAN I COPE
WITH CRPS?

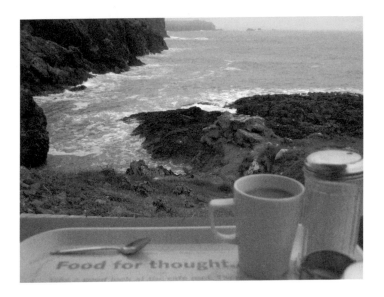

In this chapter, I take a psychological approach to try to answer this question. This is inevitable because I am a psychologist and can only write about the things I know well. Some of the following is taken from a leaflet I developed called 'Adapting to Life with CRPS'; some is drawn from my more recent practice experiences, and the rest is drawn from the published coping literature. I hope it is useful.

So, I write from the perspective of being a health psychologist. Health psychologists study ways to help people stay healthy, but, of more relevance to you, we also explore how people who are physically ill can be helped to adapt to (if chronic) or recover from (if acute) their illness. This means that we are very well suited to working with people who are living with CRPS.

Usually when I first meet someone who has CRPS, they have had quite a journey before being referred to the specialist centre in Bath. I pointed out at the start of this book that health professionals need to first rule out alternative explanations for the range of symptoms that can come with CRPS. The uncertainty that surrounds this process can be very unsettling for the person concerned and can cause them to doubt themselves. When they finally get a confirmed diagnosis of CRPS, it can bring with it a bitter-sweet feeling: they finally have an explanation for all their symptoms, but the uncertainty about prognosis, as well as frustration about how much time has passed, can be difficult to deal with. A big part of my role then as a psychologist is to help the person concerned come to terms with the difficult emotions they may be feeling and share useful ways of coping with the challenges of CRPS.

LESS EFFECTIVE COPING STRATEGIES

I have noticed that there are three common strategies people use which are not so helpful in the long term.

Denial

Some people prefer not to acknowledge that CRPS has 'happened' because acknowledging it makes it real. Talking about CRPS and the impact it is having can be difficult. Not talking about it with someone you trust can be even harder. Ignoring something does not make it go away, and indeed, for many, the attempt to ignore CRPS makes it loom ever larger.

Suffering in silence

Similarly, many people I work with have told me that although they *do* have people close to them with whom they could talk, they choose not to do so for fear of becoming 'more of a burden'. Closing off potential sources of support because you *think* you will be a burden means that you are likely to wind up coping with CRPS on your own. How do you know that you *will* be a burden? Where is the evidence for this thought? Think about how you would feel if you found out that a close friend or family member had a problem but did not turn to you because they were afraid that they would be a burden to you. How would you react? Would you feel sad that they had assumed they knew how you felt? Would you feel a little bit annoyed that, in making their decision not to talk to you, they had taken away from you the opportunity to help?

Removing self from social life

This is a sort of creeping coping strategy that happens slowly. CRPS is unpredictable and people tell me that although they make plans to attend social events, when the event actually arrives they feel they can't attend after all because their pain levels are too high and so they pull out. They tell me they begin to feel embarrassed because they assume that their friends are thinking badly of them for cancelling at the last minute. (Do you see the pattern here? They are assuming that they can read their friends' minds again, aren't they?) Instead of trusting that their real friends will understand the occasional cancellation, they feel embarrassed and begin to decline all invitations, *just in case* they need to back out at the last moment. People who choose this strategy find that their social life slowly drops away and they become more and more isolated. It might be worth thinking about this in terms of your pain. Your pain is likely to be present whether you are doing something or not. You'll be in pain whether you are at home or at a social event. Rather than being in pain, isolated and all alone at home, might it be preferable to be in pain, but be socializing with friends? A good compromise might be to accept the invitations with the caveat 'I'd love to come for a little while'; that way you are not committing yourself to the whole event or evening, but you are ensuring that you maintain your friendships and outside interests.

MORE EFFECTIVE COPING STRATEGIES

CRPS affects every area of your life; it can affect how you feel (your mood), your thoughts, your behaviour, and it can also impact on what is going on in your body. A few years ago a model was put forward by Padesky and Mooney

(1990) to show how these different areas all relate to, affect and impact on one another. You can see in Figure 3.1 how they are all connected, and so a change in one area has a knock-on effect on the others. For example, you will know that if you become stressed, perhaps your body reacts: you tense, you breathe faster and more shallowly; your heart rate speeds up. You probably also notice your feelings – perhaps fear and anxiety. Next, you notice your thoughts: 'I can't accept that invitation, I'll only let them down again'; this then feeds your tension, which feeds your negative thinking and your body's reaction and so on. Before you know it, you are in a negative spiral which leads to you turning down the invitation.

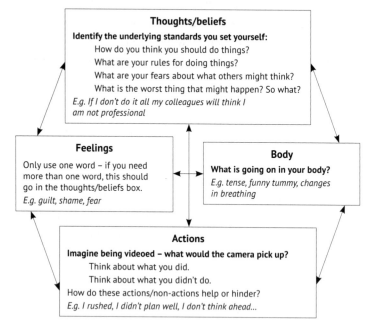

Figure 3.1: Coping model
Adapted from the Padesky and Mooney (1990) Five Part Model

Learning a range of coping strategies can help you to break the chain and, in so doing, break the downward spiral we all find ourselves in from time to time. The following sections highlight different strategies you might find helpful.

STRATEGIES TO COPE WITH BODY REACTIONS

A key skill here is to learn different relaxation techniques. What works for you may not work for someone else, so it is worth experimenting and finding out just what does work for you. For example, many people enjoy listening to relaxation recordings. If it is at all possible, I would recommend that you listen before you buy. The reason I write this is that I have at home two CDs of relaxation exercises. The script for both is identical and the exercises described are identical, and yet I can only bear to listen to one of the CDs. The only difference between the two CDs is the person narrating the exercises. One person has a voice I find relaxing; the other has a voice I cannot take seriously, and when I listen to it, I get incredibly annoyed and find the tone patronizing. Obviously, one CD is helpful for my relaxation, whereas the other has the reverse effect! As I say, the only difference between the two is the person narrating the exercises. This just shows how much personal taste can impact on us and why it is important to find something that works for you.

Similarly, many relaxation CDs will invite you to imagine yourself on a beach. The recording is likely to describe palm trees, sandy beaches and gentle waves. This vision is so far from relaxing to my taste that it does not work as an image. My ideal beach is a rocky one, perhaps just off Cornwall, with crashing waves, cold spray and lots of gusts of gale-force wind. These rugged beaches make me feel alive, in the moment and totally relaxed. I can relax into the power of nature on these kinds of beaches, whereas on a sandy hot beach I am uncomfortable and far from relaxed. The complete opposite may be true for you. This is what I mean about learning what it is that works well for you.

Before you can use relaxation strategies, it helps to learn to recognize when you are becoming stressed. This may sound like a strange thing to say, but we are generally not very good at doing this until we are very stressed indeed. When we start to pay attention to the signs our body sends us to let us know we are getting stressed, we are likely to notice the more obvious ones: perhaps our tummy feels 'funny', as if it is tied up in knots; maybe our shoulders hunch up and we 'lose our necks'; or maybe our palms get sweaty. Once we notice what our stress 'signs' are, we can put in place the relaxation strategies we have learned. As we get better at relaxation (and it takes time to master this), we also become better at reading our own signs and so are able to tune in to our stress levels earlier. The better you get at recognizing your signs, the better you will become at recognizing your stress triggers and the better equipped you will be to deal with them. So, what strategies might you try?

Visualizing a favourite place

One person I worked with vividly described her favourite place; she spoke of the heat from the sun, the song of the birds, the beauty of the room and the smell of lemons. The smell of lemons was a particularly powerful reminder for her and she now carries a little jar of lemon essential oil with her so that she can smell it whenever she wants help to retreat to her favourite place. Other people carry photographs of their favourite spots. The key to this exercise is really focusing in on your five senses. So, first choose your favourite place and think about a specific time that you were there and feeling positive. Next, think about what you could see, hear, smell, taste and feel at that time. Maybe you can see a lake, hear birdsong, smell the heather, taste the boiled sweets you were eating and feel the heat of the sun on your face. Once you have got the time, the place and your senses clear, it will be easy to visualize (imagine) this place. When you do this, you are effectively taking a mini-break from whatever it is that is stressing you.

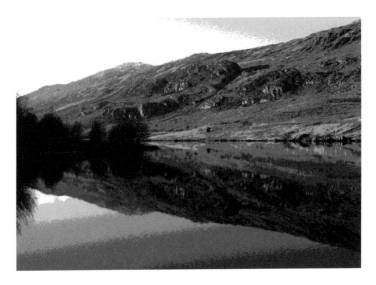

My favourite lake, Snowdonia

Breathing exercises

One technique is to focus on your breathing. Begin by choosing a word that will help you to set up your feeling of relaxation – many people use the word 'calm'. Sit as comfortably as you can, with your hands resting wherever they feel relaxed. Start breathing out slowly and let your tummy fall as you push the air out. Let your lungs fill with air again as you breathe in deeply, and notice how your tummy rises as your lungs fill.

Start counting now as you breathe out – start from 5 and steadily count down to 0 as you breathe out slowly. Then, as you breathe in, think of your chosen word (e.g. 'calm') and say it slowly in your mind. Repeat the process.

Breathe out:	5, 4, 3 ,2, 1, 0
Breathe in:	Calm
Breathe out:	5, 4, 3, 2, 1, 0
Breathe in:	Calm

Fresh air

Getting outside can help reduce tension, especially if you take a mindful walk/wheelchair ride/scooter ride, where you take time to notice all that is around you. If you are lucky enough to live near some greenery, a trip to the park can help you to feel more positive – watch the birds, look at the colours of the trees, notice the sky and so on. Getting outdoors can help you to refocus on the outside world rather than staying stuck in your internal world of worry.

STRATEGIES FOR COPING WITH FEELINGS

CRPS brings with it a whole range of feelings; common ones include anger, frustration and guilt. Holding on to these feelings only serves to increase your own stress, but it can be very hard to let go of them. Venting can help. There are a range of ways you can vent (let pent-up feelings out).

Painting

If you are in an artistic mood, you could try to paint or draw your feelings – you never know, you could end up with a masterpiece...and even if you don't, it can be a useful way of expressing how you feel.

Writing

Sometimes the best way to get the negativity out is to write down all your feelings without censoring them (yes, this can include swear words; in fact, there is research that suggests that swearing can help when coping with pain (Stephens and Umland 2011) although you will need to think about when it is appropriate to use this strategy). Take up your pen and paper (or laptop) and just let all your feelings come tumbling out. Some people find writing without a formal structure is useful – just noting down all the thoughts as and when they occur; others find that a more structured approach helps – perhaps writing poetry. Many people find that when they have finished writing, tearing up the paper into small pieces and throwing it away helps to symbolically throw away the negative thoughts and feelings.

Keeping diaries

It can be difficult for you to recognize the progress you make when you are in the midst of change. One way to help you notice your progress is to keep a diary. This way, when you look back, you can remember what it used to be like and will find it easier to identify the things you find you are now able to do that you weren't before. When you write in your diary, be sure to remember to actively look for and to include the positive things that happen each day.

Even on a bad day, it *is* possible to find something good that happened. This can be as simple as managing to get up at the time you planned, even though you felt awful, or maybe someone held a door open for you. Looking for, noticing and writing about the positive things sounds like a simple strategy, but it really does lift your mood. The diary will also help you to monitor your progress. It can be easy to forget the progress you make – because we are human beings we are always focused on the next thing and often forget to celebrate the achievements along the way.

Acknowledging the feeling

A simple technique is to just name the feeling: 'Oh, I'm feeling guilty', 'Oh, I'm feeling angry', 'Oh, I'm feeling frustrated'. Naming a feeling helps us to look at it more objectively and to question and explore what might be going on behind the feeling. It *is* OK to have negative feelings; there is no rule that says we should be 'chipper' all the time. You were not always positive and happy before you were diagnosed with CRPS; why, then, should things be different now? Acknowledge the feeling, try to understand what is driving it and work out whether there is anything you can do about it. If yes, do something. If not, recognize that the feeling *will* pass.

Humour as support

Some people develop a black sense of humour which they find helps them to cope. One person I worked with developed a supportive relationship with two other women who also had CRPS. They called themselves the 'Raspberry Ripples' (rhyming slang for 'cripple') and had a theme tune – 'I Don't Feel Like Dancin'' by the Scissor Sisters. This person described how the use of humour helped her and her friends to support one another and maintain morale.

STRATEGIES FOR DEALING WITH THOUGHTS

Thoughts are fleeting things – they come of their own accord and there is little we can do to stop them coming. What we can do, however, is stop listening to them. I heard someone wise once say, 'You can't stop the thoughts from coming, but you *can* stop inviting them to stay for a cup of tea.' Many of the thoughts we have are ones we have time and time again – they are habitual ways of thinking. Our inner voice is what we hear, and that voice is often negative and critical. For example, 'I can't believe you said that; now they will all know you are stupid' is a common thought most of us have experienced at one time or another. What can happen is that the more often we have a thought, the more likely we are to begin to believe it. The more we believe in it, the more thoughts can influence emotions, and we can descend in a negative downward spiral. This can then colour our view of the world.

If we can learn to recognize our habitual ways of thinking, we can begin to question them and hold them up to scrutiny. How true is that thought? Where is the evidence for that thought? If we stick with the example above – 'I can't believe you said that, now they will all know you are stupid' – and question it, what we often find is that the thought might be true of a specific situation or event, but it is not something that is representative of who we are. So you may well have said something thoughtless or silly, but this does not mean that you as a person are stupid. Learning to recognize these thought patterns and to both question *and* seek evidence for the truth of the thought will help you to avoid getting stuck on the downward spiral.

Rules (musts / shoulds)

Many of us have unwritten rules by which we live our lives. These may have worked for you prior to CRPS, but often these rules are unhelpful and become another means of 'beating yourself up' by trying to live up to an ideal of how you think things *should* be, rather than working with how things *are*. Whenever you catch yourself saying 'I must' or 'I should', it is a sure sign that there is a rule driving this thought and, consequently, your behaviour. Again, use the questioning technique. Ask yourself why you should or why you must do whatever it is. Is the rule something you have imposed on yourself? Ask yourself what would happen if you did not do this thing and think about whether there might be different ways of doing whatever it is.

Acceptance

This is definitely not an easy concept, but the process of coming to terms with, and accepting your illness and your new identity can provide you with a sense of closure. It is ultimately a more positive step, because rather than grieving for the loss of your pre-CRPS self, in accepting your illness you are then able to begin moving forward.

The other thing to remember is that you don't have to do it alone. Try to give others a chance to help you. Learn practical tips on how to manage your symptoms and emotions on a daily basis. Seek out things that you can enjoy. Find your 'heroes' or people who are coping successfully with disabling and painful conditions, and learn from them. Focus on looking for the positive and on the things that you *can* do.

People trying to cope with CRPS sometimes fear that acceptance of CRPS amounts to giving in. Acceptance is not a bad thing. It does not mean that you have given up fighting or that you are inviting CRPS to stay with you for ever. What acceptance can do, however, is change your focus to one which looks towards making the most of your current abilities and living in the present, rather than being stuck in the past and wishing things were different.

Suicidal thoughts

It is relatively common for people to experience thoughts relating to suicide when coping with a chronic painful condition. These thoughts can be passive – 'I'd happily go to sleep and not wake up' or 'Sometimes I wish it were all over' – or active – 'I've thought about just ending it all.' These thoughts do not necessarily mean that a person is suicidal, nor are they an indicator of the severity of the problem. What they do show is that the person experiencing these thoughts is very distressed and struggling.

Suicidal thoughts are always upsetting and problematic for the person experiencing them and they must always be taken seriously. If you are having suicidal thoughts, it is extremely important that you talk to someone about how you are feeling. If you can, speak to a family member or friend, or your GP. If you have a current therapist or psychiatrist, tell them how you are feeling. If you don't feel that you can speak to someone face to face, call the Samaritans on 08457 909090 – they are an excellent non-judgemental listening service.

Crisis card

When your pain is particularly bad, or you feel especially down, angry or sad, it can be hard to remember the strategies you could engage in that may help you to feel better. It can be hard to see out of the black hole you find yourself in. At these times it can be really helpful to have a crisis card to hand. It is a good idea to make this card at a time when you are feeling relatively positive. On this card, you write down the things you can do and list the people you can turn to (along with their telephone numbers) when you are in crisis. You could also include helpline numbers (e.g. Samaritans), things you can do to distract yourself, perhaps paint, write, read, watch a DVD, listen to a relaxation CD and so on...whatever works for you (see Figure 3.2). Once you have written your strategies on the card, you simply pop it in your purse or wallet and you will have it with you, ready for the next time you feel especially down and can't think how best to cope.

Listen to music

Go for a walk

Take a bath

Light Incense

Meditate

Telephone sister(s)

Figure 3.2: Example crisis card

On the other side of the card, you could put a photograph of your favourite place, so the card also works as a means of relaxation – you can focus on the photograph and take yourself to this special place. In doing so you can escape your world for a while.

BEHAVIOURAL STRATEGIES

This section is about what you do, and, indeed, what you don't do, out of habit. Again, key to this is bringing to your awareness your habitual ways of responding and exploring whether these responses are still useful. You will find suggestions below to help you to think about different ways of behaving in response to different situations.

Stock story

People living with CRPS tell me that when someone asks what is wrong with them, although they don't want to, they feel they should explain CRPS in detail. Many people find that saying 'I have CRPS' is not enough. This is because so few people have heard of the condition and are keen to ask more questions (What is CRPS? How did you get it? Is it catching?). One way to address this problem is to develop a 'stock story'.

For example, one person I worked with had CRPS in her foot and needed to alter her position regularly. As a result, she could not sit or stand for long periods of time. However, she found it difficult to explain this to people she was meeting for the first time at work events. On previous occasions, she had said nothing because she did not wish to be viewed as different or as less capable than her colleagues. After some discussion with her, she agreed to try out the phrase, 'I have a problem with my foot and I need to alternate walking around with sitting down.' She was amazed at its simplicity – there was no need to go into lots of detail about CRPS; all she needed to do was to state her needs clearly. Other people simply say that they have a 'rare form of arthritis'. They tell me that because people have heard of arthritis and know how painful it can be, they don't ask lots of follow-up questions.

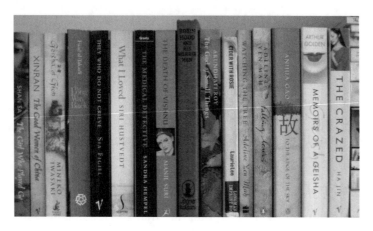

What's your story?

Pacing

Pacing is about achieving the right balance between different types of exertion and rest periods. We all find this difficult to do. Ask anyone how they are nowadays and the typical response is 'busy'. We are all squeezing too much into too small an amount of time and space. This is not a good strategy when we are well, but when we are learning to live with a chronic condition, such as CRPS, pacing becomes hugely important – after all, we are human beings, *not* human doings! So how do you go about managing your precious energy levels? Author Virginia Haydon outlines the following:

Establish a routine: One aim of pacing is to make activity and rest patterns more consistent. It's all about staying within energy limits without over- or under-activity.

Work out what's right for you: It can be helpful to plan the same amount of activity and the same amount of rest every day. For this reason it is crucial to set your initial activity levels within your own personal comfort zone. They must reflect what you are already doing, not what you wish you could do. Try to recognize that tasks such as getting washed and dressed are physical and should not be underestimated.

Set clear goals: Writing down your goals will make it easier to fix them in your mind. Specific daily targets according to your energy levels might include getting up and going to bed at the same time or walking for 'x' minutes per day. It's worth remembering that emotions take their toll on energy levels too. That's why we feel so exhausted after a long hard cry. Remember that the goals that are right for you are likely to be different for another person with CRPS. There is no standard map.

Organization and planning: Setting yourself a programme of rest and activity periods throughout the day is one thing; sticking to it is the hard bit. It helps if you plan your week ahead as well as each day, making a note of what you want to achieve and then prioritizing what matters most to you.

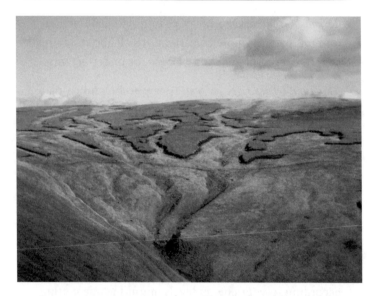

There is no standard map: A map of the world or just the
way the peat arranged itself in the Brecon Beacons?

Remember to allow sufficient time to complete tasks.
There is immense satisfaction at being able to tick off
a successfully achieved task, no matter how simple.
Being overambitious only leads to disappointment
and frustration. If things are going well, don't be
tempted to do more than you planned, particularly on
a good day. Likewise, don't be too disappointed if you
are faced with a setback.

Also, don't forget that just because you have
been organized and planned your time and activities,
it does not mean that life will go along with your
plans. It didn't work like this before you had CRPS
and it won't work like that now. As you are very well
aware, life throws up unexpected situations and being
flexible can help you overcome them without your
schedule disintegrating before your eyes. (Haydon
2004, pp.22–23)

Videos

Some people have found that videoing themselves as they perform their exercises, such as walking, can be useful because it helps them to see the progress that they have made. However, be aware that the first time you see yourself on video can be a surprise – very much like the first time you hear your voice on tape.

Accessing and accepting support

At times it can be difficult to access the support we need. It is important to learn how to communicate our needs to those around us. No matter how much someone loves us, we cannot expect them to be able to read our minds. Unless we tell them what we need or what we want, how can we possibly expect them to be able to guess? This means that one of the key skills you will need to develop is that of communicating your needs to those around you.

However, before you can communicate what your needs are, it can be helpful to take some time to be clear in your mind just what it is you need. With CRPS, it can be all too easy to become completely focused on your pain at the expense of all other aspects of your life. One way to take an objective look at the balance in your life is to draw up two 'life grids' – one for your life pre-CRPS and one for your life as it is now. Include as many boxes as you need. In each box, you record an important aspect of your life. This may include people who are important to you, activities you enjoy doing, pets you have and so on.

An example might look like Figure 3.3:

Before CRPS

Partner	Swimming	Choir
Friends	Going to the pub	Playing with the kids
Cooking	Walking the dog	Eating out

After CRPS

Pain	Partner

Figure 3.3: Life grid exercise

You can see that the second grid is very much smaller than the first. This person's life has contracted as their focus has become directed on their pain. Once you can see clearly how the balance of your life has changed, you will then be able to work out the kind of support you might need and the direction you might need to take to help you to develop a better balance and focus for your life. One person I worked with called this process 'Putting life first and CRPS second'.

For example, it might not be possible to engage in the sports you used to, but there might be other sports that are now more suitable for your current level of mobility (e.g. fishing, archery, swimming). Alternatively, you may be able to stay involved with your hobby of choice, but be involved in a different way. One lady who used to show dogs was no longer able to carry on breeding and showing dogs, but she really missed the shows. She began to think about how she could stay involved. She remembered that she still had contact details for other breeders and decided that she would offer to help them when they were taking part in dog shows. This meant that she could stay involved with an activity she loved, in a way that matched her current level of physical ability.

There is no doubt that engaging in this 'life grid' exercise requires a considerable amount of bravery on your part, but rebalancing your life can be very rewarding and helps you as you redefine who you are now and what your current needs are.

Communication

I have noticed that many of the people living with CRPS who I work with communicate in what is called a 'passive' way. Passive communication is when you don't express your feelings, needs, rights and opinions, but focus your attention on the other person's feelings, needs, rights and opinions. This is often driven by the feeling the person with CRPS has of being a 'burden'. Fearing that you are a burden makes you hide your true feelings and needs. The problem with this is that your needs are then not met and you can begin to feel worse about yourself and even less likely to ask for whatever it is you need. Before you know it, you are in a downward spiral.

Passive communication can cause frustration to build up, which might lead to you communicating in an aggressive way. This is almost the opposite of passive in that you stop thinking about the other person's needs and only express your feelings in what might be an angry and demanding way. This kind of communication doesn't help either and also leads to you feeling bad about yourself. Handily, there is a middle way and it is a way which, if you can master it, will keep you calm, even in difficult situations. This is especially important for people living with CRPS, because an increase in stress often leads to an increase in pain. This middle way is called communicating assertively.

Communicating assertively is all about respecting your needs, feelings, rights and opinions (as well as those of the other person). In other words, you will move yourself higher up your list of priorities – *your needs matter too.*

Initially, this can be quite hard to do, but those who have mastered the technique say that at the start they *acted as if* they felt their needs mattered, and eventually began to *really feel* that their needs mattered. One thing to note is that you will not always remember to use this strategy. You are a human being, and therefore I am sorry to tell you that you are not perfect – none of us are! In short, there are three key parts to communicating assertively. I use a simple model which I know as the A, B, C of communication.

1. *Listening to others.* If you think about a time when you have been in conversation with someone who only talked about themselves, you will remember how annoying it is. Not being heard or listened to by someone is very annoying. So the first step in communicating assertively is to show the other person that you have heard them. You do not need to agree with what they are saying, but you do need to acknowledge their opinion. [**A = Acknowledge**]

2. *Say how you feel.* Telling someone how you feel is important. The other person cannot argue with you – they cannot say that you do not feel something. In telling them how you feel, you should put your point of view across briefly and without apologizing. So you begin by acknowledging the other person and then you say, 'But this is how I feel.' [**B = But**]

3. *Finding a way forward together.* By being open to working collaboratively, you might find some middle ground, a new solution or a way of blending both your positions. [**C = Compromise**]

SUMMARY

So, the eagle-eyed amongst you will have noticed that I structured this section of the book around the four issues of the model I introduced at the start of this chapter: body, feelings, thoughts and behaviours. In some ways, it is a little fake to split things up in this way because all of these things are very interlinked. I think that the take-home message underlying this chapter is that much of what we do, we do without thinking. This means that we spend a lot of our time reacting to situations in a habitual way, rather than taking time to step back and trying to evaluate the situation. *Catching thoughts and negative thinking habits* – assuming we know what others think ('They'll think I'm a burden') and catastrophizing (assuming the worst) – is an important skill to develop because these kinds of thoughts and habitual ways of responding to situations can have a huge impact on how we behave and how our body reacts. It is also important to give yourself and those around you some slack. We are all human and none of us is perfect.

This message was brought home to me recently when I bumped into a group of people on our two-week rehabilitation programme who had nipped to Waitrose for treats at the end of the day to celebrate their progress. They regaled me with an incident that had happened earlier that day. Four of them had CRPS in their legs and one had CRPS in his arm. The group had been engaged in banter and one had in jest punched another on his (CRPS-affected) arm. She said she realized her mistake immediately and tried to put it right by rubbing his arm, thereby making the situation even worse. The person whose arm had been punched told me that he had just about coped with the punch, but that the rubbing had almost 'sent him through the roof'. Although they were laughing when telling the story, I thought it a really useful tale because it highlights that even people with CRPS forget – so perhaps we should not be so hard when family, friends and work colleagues also forget.

I think that a key skill for learning to cope with CRPS is to look actively for things that work for you. Listen to other people in other situations and contexts and see if adapting what they do might be helpful for you. Useful suggestions can come from unexpected sources. By way of example, I was working with someone who had isolated herself from friends and family and had begun to choose not to answer the door when friends and family visited – therefore isolating herself even more. When we were talking, she said that she did not like doing this, but that she found it hard to tell visitors that she would prefer to catch up with them at a different time – as a consequence, she was ignoring her doorbell. I remembered a piece of advice that had been given by the presenter Graham Norton on a radio show and I shared it with my client. Mr Norton had said that he puts on a coat before he answers his door. Doing this gives him the opportunity to answer the door and decide whether he wants to spend time with the person who is there. If he does not, he simply says he was just on his way out and suggests they catch up another time. If, on the other hand, he is happy to spend time with the unexpected visitor, he is able to say that he had just got in and invites the person in. The coat enables him to manage this situation. This simple strategy caught the imagination of the person I was working with and she felt more confident in her ability to cope because she now had a feeling of being in control of the situation.

Finally, the suggestions in this section of the book are just that – suggestions. Some will resonate with you and others are things that you will instinctively reject because they are not things you can see yourself doing. This is fine. The message is to find something that works for you and use it.

Chapter 4

CRPS DOES NOT JUST AFFECT THE PERSON WHO IS DIAGNOSED WITH CRPS

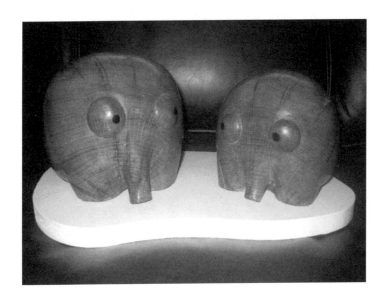

When you are in the midst of coming to terms with CRPS and all the different ways it is affecting you, it can be very hard to recognize that CRPS also affects those around you, especially loved ones, friends and family.

It can be very difficult for your loved ones because they see at close quarters just how hard it is for you to cope with all the challenges that come with CRPS, and it is all the more difficult for them because it can feel as if all they can do is stand by helplessly, wishing they could do something. Your friends, family and loved ones can feel just as frustrated and angry as you do about CRPS.

Your friends, family and loved ones can play an important role in supporting you, if you let them and if you find a way to work together. This will involve you recognizing that they are also affected by CRPS and you each learning to speak honestly, kindly and clearly to one another. All too often I hear a person with CRPS telling me that if their partner *really loved them*, they would *know* how to help. After a consultation with a person with CRPS, I am often taken to one side by the partner who tells me that they don't know how to help because their partner won't talk about CRPS. It is important to remember that we are just human beings; we are not mind readers and the only way we can ever know what someone else wants is (a) if they tell us or (b) if we ask them. Sounds simple, doesn't it? But it seems to be a difficult skill to master.

We know from research done in other fields that involving carers (I'll use this term to mean friends, family and loved ones) can maximize the benefits of rehabilitation (e.g. Carr and Shepherd 1987) and can help people to maintain the gains that they make in rehabilitation (e.g. Evans *et al.* 1994). We as a team wanted to learn more about the experiences of the carers of people we had seen at the hospital and so we interviewed ten carers. We wrote our research up and published it in an academic journal (Lauder *et al.* 2011), but I will summarize the main points here in the hope that you find them useful.

We found that the carers were really keen to try to understand the experiences that their relative or friend was going through and put a lot of effort into trying to understand CRPS *and* the rehabilitation process. It was clear during the interviews that CRPS had very much become a part of their lives too.

Making sense of CRPS

In an earlier study (Rodham, McCabe and Blake 2009), we reported that people with CRPS felt that no one else could ever truly understand what it was like to have CRPS unless they had it themselves. Whilst it is true that none of us can ever fully understand how things are for another person, it *is* possible to have insight and empathy for what another person is going through. In the case of the carers we interviewed, it was very clear that they recognized that CRPS pain was real and at times unbearable. They struggled to find words that they thought fully captured the pain experience of their loved ones, but, in trying to find the right words, they revealed a depth of understanding and empathy for the person they were trying to support. They felt that their ability to understand and learn about CRPS was vital for them to be able to help their relative or friend. As such, they were also spending a lot of time actively seeking information and trying to make sense of what they felt was a mysterious condition. Gleaning information from the internet was not an easy task and what they found made them feel terribly anxious; the information was often complex and fear-provoking because they came across worst-case scenarios.

Being in tune with the person with CRPS

The carers in our study were highly tuned in to the physical and emotional needs of their loved one. They spoke of watching and looking for signs of distress, and in fact explained how they had learned to interpret the non-verbal behaviour of their friend or relative. They saw this as important because they were well aware that their loved one was making an effort to hide just how much pain they were in. So, a sort of unspoken agreement had happened over time where the carer would monitor the person with CRPS and the environment, keeping an eye out for potential pain triggers so that they could shield their loved one.

Role of protector

As such, the carer often took on the role of protector – trying to keep a safe zone around the person with CRPS. Although on some levels this was helpful, because it gave them a sense that they were doing something useful, it can have negative impacts for both the person with CRPS and the carer themselves. Monitoring and protecting, although done with good intent, can take away the independence of the person with CRPS, and can make them lose confidence in their ability to deal with normal everyday situations. Indeed, a key element of successful coping with CRPS is taking responsibility for one's own behaviour or reactions to difficult situations. If you have a well-meaning carer doing this for you, you can relinquish more responsibility and independence, which in turn has a negative impact on how you feel.

Taking on the role of protector can also have negative consequences for the carer. Initially, it might feel good to be playing an active role in helping their loved one to cope with CRPS – but, in the long term, they might be contributing to the person living with CRPS becoming overdependent on them; in the shorter term, taking on such a big responsibility – monitoring and protecting – is exhausting. Carers may find that their own energy levels and coping resources become depleted. If a carer is spending all their energy on their loved one, they will have no energy left for their own needs.

Understanding rehabilitation

Most of the carers we spoke to hoped that a cure for CRPS would be found. This hope can lead to unrealistic expectations of rehabilitation programmes, which in turn can lead to disappointment. A rehabilitation programme focuses on improving physical function, not cure (at present there is no cure). It was clear that the message about what might be realistic expectations to hold had not always filtered through to the carers. There is perhaps a need for an information resource to be developed that is directed at carers.

Supporting rehabilitation

The carers we spoke to found it difficult to judge how far to push their loved one on their return home. One talked about a fine line between encouragement and nagging. It was also hard for them to encourage their loved ones to do the exercises and desensitization when it was clear that their loved one's pain was increasing. It was a difficult position to be in – encouraging their loved one to persevere with painful processes.

Working together

Attending appointments with their loved one was something carers valued because they felt better informed and, as a consequence of this, felt better able to provide support. This was especially valued with regard to the physiotherapy appointments where carers could observe the physiotherapist modelling how to support and encourage someone to do the exercises even when they were in pain.

SUMMARY

So, what was really clear from this study was that CRPS had also become very much a part of the carers' own lives as they tried to monitor, protect and motivate their loved ones. Witnessing the pain experienced by the person with CRPS meant that carers tried to do whatever they could to minimize their loved ones' distress. They were keen to learn more about CRPS and about how they could best help their loved ones.

BUT...

So far we have explored how CRPS impacts on the carer's ability to support the person with CRPS. It is also important to spend some time recognizing and focusing on how CRPS might impact on the carers themselves.

Carers also experience losses. Their life is also affected and changed by the introduction of CRPS. It can be frustrating for them – their future plans are also taken away from them. They might feel that the person with CRPS has no understanding of how things are for them, and it can be a difficult issue to raise because they feel that they are being selfish just by giving voice to their experiences. How can it be OK for them to say how difficult things are for them when they are not the ones who have been diagnosed with CRPS?

It is important to remember that *it is not a competition* to see whose life has been most or worst affected. Often what is needed is an acknowledgement from the person with CRPS that things are both difficult and different for everyone.

So how can carers help themselves to cope?

Make sure you have a *good support network* and make sure that you use it. It is OK to feel angry, frustrated, sad, fed up (sometimes all at once) about the situation that you and your loved one find yourselves in. Make sure you have someone to talk to about how you are feeling. If you don't have someone close, then think about talking to a professional (you could ask your GP for recommendations).

Make sure you *keep your own interests going* – doing so will help you to keep a level of normality in your life as you and your loved one adjust to life with CRPS.

Become informed – seek information. Ask health professionals where you can get hold of information that they consider to be sound. There is a lot of unpleasant and simply wrong information online; get help to find that which is both useful and 'evidence-based'.

Talk to your loved one honestly about how you are feeling and about how they feel you can best support them (and they you). Communication is key and it is a good idea to stop second-guessing what your loved one might be thinking and instead work together to find a system of coping that works for you both.

Remember that *your needs are just as important as those of your loved one.* If you are taking on more of a supportive role, you will need to remember to look after yourself too. Imagine yourself as a jug of water. Each time you provide/offer support you are essentially pouring some of your water into the other person's glass; eventually, your jug will be empty and you will have nothing left to give. In other words, you need to keep yourself topped up. How you might do this will be different for each person – it might be through your hobbies, sports and/or socializing. Keep doing whatever it is that gives you 'you time' and keeps you topped up.

How can the person with CRPS help their loved one to cope?

It is a two-way street this support business. I think that key for the person with CRPS is to remember to take a step back every now and then. It is very easy (we all do this) to only see things from our own point of view. When we do this, we are blinded to alternative perspectives, and as a result you might forget that CRPS is an issue for your loved one too – check in with them every now and then to see how they are feeling. Working together in partnership with friends, family and loved ones will make adapting to life with CRPS a smoother journey.

Chapter 5

ENDINGS...

So, we come to the end of this book. Inevitably, I have presented a biased view throughout – this biased view of mine is coloured by my psychological training and the experiences I have had of both working with people living with CRPS and researching how people cope with the challenges of CRPS.

I have briefly covered what CRPS is, how it is diagnosed and treated. More importantly, the biggest part of the focus of this book has been on sharing real people's stories about living with CRPS and on strategies to cope with CRPS. I have also included a section for those who are the friends and family of people living with CRPS – a group that is often neglected.

I could try to draw out some concluding points, but I think that it is better to leave it for you to draw your own conclusions. This is not a book designed to give you neat answers, for there are none. Instead, I have attempted to share some of the lessons I have learned over the past six or seven years in the hope that they will be a useful resource for people who are living with and learning to live with CRPS, as well as for their friends and family.

I wish you all well on your individual journeys as you learn to cope with the challenges that come with CRPS. I sincerely hope that you do manage to achieve the goal of putting life first and CRPS second.

USEFUL RESOURCES

GENERAL
Breathworks
Provides courses, products and training in mindfulness-based pain and illness management. The site has tips and resources about relaxation and mindfulness.

> Website: www.breathworks-mindfulness.org.uk

Karen Rodham's website
Contains links to leaflets and CRPS information.

> Website: https://sites.google.com/site/profkarenrodham

UK
British Association for Counselling and Psychotherapy (BACP)
BACP aims to increase public understanding of the benefits of counselling and psychotherapy, raise awareness of what can be expected from the process of therapy, and promote education and/or training for counsellors and psychotherapists. They can refer people to a local counsellor.

> Website: www.bacp.co.uk

Carers UK
Carers UK provides information, advice and support for carers. By bringing carers together, they campaign to make life better for carers and influence policy makers, employers and service providers, to help them improve carers' lives.

> Website: www.carersuk.org

British Complementary Medical Association

Can give names of registered therapists, and advice on what to look for in a complementary therapist.

Website: www.bcma.co.uk

CRPS UK Clinical and Research Network

Aims to raise awareness and understanding of CRPS amongst health professionals, patients and the general public.

Website: www.crpsnetworkuk.org

CRPS Community

Made by a person with CRPS for people with CRPS.

Website: www.crpscommunity.co.uk

CRPSUK

An email list for those in the UK who are diagnosed with CRPS. Send an email to this address and join the mailing list.

Email: adm-crpsuk@hotmail.com

Mind

An organization which aims to make sure anyone with a mental health problem has somewhere to turn to for advice and support.

Website: www.mind.org.uk

Royal College of Physicians

UK guidelines for diagnosis, referral and management in primary and secondary care.

Website: www.rcplondon.ac.uk/sites/default/files/documents/complex-regional-pain-full-guideline.pdf

Samaritans

Available 24 hours a day to provide confidential emotional support for people who are experiencing feelings of distress, despair or suicidal thoughts.

Tel: 08457 909090

Website: www.samaritans.co.uk

USA

American RSDHope

Run by volunteers who are either patients or who have a loved one who is. They aim to raise awareness of CRPS/RSD.

Website: www.rsdhope.org

Lehigh Valley RSD/CRPS Support Group

Run by people who are living with RSD/CRPS with the aim of supporting patients diagnosed with RSD/CRPS. They also aim to educate and advocate for patients and their caregivers, as well as actively promoting public and professional awareness of RSD/CRPS.

Website: https://sites.google.com/site/lvrsdcrpssupportgroup/

Email: lvrsdcrps@gmail.com

Power of Pain Foundation (POPF)

A not-for-profit charity that provides community-based support services that address needs of chronic pain patients with neuropathy conditions such as RSD/CRPS.

Website: http://powerofpain.org

Reflex Sympathetic Dystrophy Association (RSDA)

The mission of this organization is to provide support, education and hope to everyone affected by CRPS/RSD while driving research to develop better treatment and a cure.

Website: www.rsds.org

RSD Awareness

Created by parents and grandparents with children or grandchildren who have RSD/CRPS. Their goal is to raise awareness and to provide support for those living with RSD/CRPS.

Website: www.rsdawareness.com

Email: admin@rsdawareness.com

Rocky Mountain CRPS/RSD (RMRSD)

Rocky Mountain CRPS/RSD is a registered non-profit organization run by an all-volunteer board of directors. Their primary focus is to raise money for CRPS research. They also provide education and support services to the CRPS community at large.

Website: www.rmrsd.org

Tel: (303) 918-9385

Triumph Over Pain

A non-profit organization working to further education, raise awareness and increase research on pain diseases by uniting the pain community, teaming with the medical professional community, the general public and those affected by chronic pain to bring about awareness, understanding and cooperation within these communities.

Website: www.triumphoverpain.org

AUSTRALIA

The Australian Reflex Sympathetic Dystrophy Support Group

A site run by people who are themselves living with CRPS/RSD. They aim to provide information and support for those living with CRPS/RSD.

Website: www.ozrsd.org

The Australian RSD/CRPS Support Group

Run by a person who is living with CRPS/RSD, offering information and support for others living with CRPS/RSD.

Website: http://australianrsdcrps.webs.com

Email: australianrsdcrps@gmail.com

Chronic Pain Australia

Run by a group of volunteers including people in pain, researchers, health professionals and advocates who work towards destigmatizing chronic pain. Their aim is to provide high-quality user-friendly research-based information and support via an online forum.

Website: www.chronicpainaustralia.org.au

CANADA

Chronic Pain Association of Canada

The Chronic Pain Association of Canada is an independent, not-for-profit charitable organization serving people affected by pain through education, information and support advocacy. They describe themselves as 'a grass roots organization that has grown because of a desperate need for relief of chronic pain'.

Website: http://chronicpaincanada.com

Promoting Awareness of RSD and CRPS in Canada (PARC)

PARC is a registered charity. Its mission is to support, educate and inform those with RSD/CRPS, the community and the medical professionals treating RSD. They also fund research into CRPS/RSD.

Website: www.rsdcanada.org

INTERNATIONAL

International Association for the Study of Pain

Founded in 1973, IASP is the world's largest multidisciplinary organization focused specifically on pain research and treatment.

Website: www.iasp-pain.org

USEFUL BOOKS

Two wonderfully written books about depression: one written for the person with depression, and the other for friends and family of someone living with depression:

Johnstone, M. (2007) *I Had a Black Dog.* London: Constable and Robinson.

Johnston, M. and Johnstone, A. (2008) *Living with a Black Dog.* London: Constable and Robinson.

A really useful book teaching us how to catch our thoughts and turn them round:

Van Bilson, H. (2009) *Zee Beatty and The Socks of Doom.* Hertford: The Cognitive Behavioural Therapy Partnership.

A book about relaxation, meditation and quieting those noisy and unwelcome thoughts we all experience from time to time:

Johnstone, M. (2011) *Quiet the Mind*. London: Constable and Robinson.

A story about learning to be kind to yourself – something we should all do! It is a children's story with a powerful message and one I use in my teaching at university as well as in my practice as a psychologist:

Reynolds, P.H. (2004) *Ish*. Somerville, MA: Candlewick Press.

REFERENCES

Baron, R., Fields, H.L., Jänig, W., Kitt, C. and Levine, J.D. (2002) 'National Institutes of Health Workshop: Reflex sympathetic dystrophy/complex regional pain syndromes – state-of-the-science.' *Anesthesia and Analgesia 95*, 6, 1812–1816.

Carr, J.H. and Shepherd, R.B. (1987) *A Motor Relearning Programme for Stroke* (2nd edition). Oxford: Heinemann Medical Books.

De Mos, M., Huygen, F.J.P.M., van der Hoeven-Borgman, M., Dieleman, J.P., Ch Stricker, B.H. and Sturkenboom, M.C. (2009) 'Outcome of the complex regional pain syndrome.' *Clinical Journal of Pain 25*, 7, 590–597.

Evans, R.L., Connis, R.T., Bishop, D.S., Hendricks, R.D. and Haselkorn, J.K. (1994) 'Stroke: A family dilemma.' *Disability Rehabilitation 16*, 3, 110–118.

Galer, B.B., Henderson, J., Perander, J. and Jensen, M.P. (2000) 'Course of symptoms and quality of life measurement in complex regional pain syndrome: A pilot survey.' *Journal of Pain Symptom Management 20*, 4, 286–292.

Goebel, A., Barker, C.H., Turner-Stokes, L. *et al.* (2012) *Complex Regional Pain Syndrome in Adults: UK Guidelines for Diagnosis, Referral and Management in Primary and Secondary Care.* London: RCP.

Harden, R.N. (2001) 'Complex regional pain syndrome.' *British Journal of Anaesthesia 87*, 1, 99–106.

Harden, R.N., Bruehl, S., Perez, R.S., Birklein, F. *et al.* (2010) 'Validation of proposed diagnostic criteria (the "Budapest criteria") for complex regional pain syndrome.' *Pain 150*, 2, 268–274.

Haydon, V. (2004) 'Pacing: One step at a time.' *Talking Point 2*, 22–23.

Kozin, F. (2005) 'Reflex Sympathetic Dystrophy.' In D.J. Wallace and D.J. Clauw (eds) *Fibromyalgia and Other Central Pain Syndromes.* Philadelphia, PA: Lippincott Williams and Wilkins.

Lauder, A., McCabe, C., Rodham, K. and Norris, E. (2011) 'An exploration of the support person's perceptions and experiences of complex regional pain syndrome and the rehabilitation process.' *Musculoskeletal Care 9,* 3, 169–179.

Lewis, J.S., Kersten, P., McCabe, C.S., McPherson, K.M. and Blake, D.R. (2007) 'Body perception disturbance: A contribution to pain in complex regional pain syndrome (CRPS).' *Pain 133,* 1–3, 111–119.

Lohnberg, J.A. and Altmaier, E.M. (2013) 'A review of psychosocial factors in complex regional pain syndrome.' *Journal of Clinical Psychology in Medical Settings 20,* 2, 247–254.

McBride, A. and Atkins, B. (2005) 'Complex regional pain syndrome.' *Current Orthopaedics 19,* 2, 155–165.

Padesky, C.A. and Mooney, K.A. (1990) 'Clinical tip: Presenting the cognitive model to clients.' *International Cognitive Therapy Newsletter 6,* 13–14.

Rodham, K., McCabe, C. and Blake, D. (2009) 'Seeking support: An interpretative phenomenological analysis of an internet message board for people with complex regional pain syndrome.' *Psychology and Health 24,* 6, 619–634.

Stanton-Hicks, M. (2006) 'Complex regional pain syndrome: Manifestations and the role of neuro-stimulation in its management.' *Journal of Pain Symptom Management 31,* 4S, S20–24.

Stanton-Hicks, M., Jänig, W., Hassenbusch, S., Haddox, J.D., Boas, R. and Wilson, P. (1995) 'Reflex sympathetic dystrophy: Changing concepts and taxonomy.' *Pain 63,* 1, 127–133.

Stephens, R. and Umland, C. (2011) 'Swearing as a response to pain: Effect of daily swearing frequency.' *The Journal of Pain 12,* 12, 1274–1281.

Veldman, P.J., Reynen, H.M., Arntz, I.E. and Goris, R.J. (1993) 'Signs and symptoms of reflex sympathetic dystrophy: Prospective study of 829 patients.' *Lancet 342,* 8878, 1012–1016.

INDEX

Page references in *italic* indicate Figures.

abandonment fears 20
acceptance 30, 31, 43, 64–5, 90, 106–7
anger 91, 102
anxiety 63, 67, 80
    about health 72–3, 81
    over treatment 20
    and the Padesky and Mooney coping
        model 98
    panic attacks 41
    see also fear
assertiveness 115–16

Bath CPRS centre and rehabilitation
    programme 27, 34, 87, 95
behaviour
    behavioural strategies 34, 49, 62,
        63–4, 90, 109–16
    communicative *see* communication
    and the Padesky and Mooney coping
        model 98
beliefs
    and the Padesky and Mooney coping
        model 98
    repeated thoughts giving rise to 105
body perception disturbance (BPD) 19
body reactions
    negative feelings towards affected part
        of body 55, 60, 77, 82–3
    and the Padesky and Mooney coping
        model 98
    recognizing signs and triggers of stress
        100
    strategies to cope with 99–102
BPD (body perception disturbance) 19
breathing exercises 101–2
Budapest Criteria 16

carers 123–9
    being in tune with the person with
        CRPS 125
    and communication 128
    energy levels 126
    getting correct information about
        CRPS 124–5, 128
    helping themselves to cope 128–9
    protector role 125–6
    and rehabilitation 123–4, 126–7
    sense of loss 127–8
    support network 128
    working together with 58, 127, 129
communication
    assertive 115–16
    A, B, C model 116
    carer information and education
        124–5, 128
    between carers and a person with
        CRPS 128
    with family 36, 53, 55, 70, 107
    of feelings 36, 115–16
    internet information/searches on
        CRPS 20–21, 28, 40, 53, 66–7,
        70, 81, 124–5
    and listening 116
    with others who also have CRPS 36,
        50, 77–8
    passive 115
    patient information *see* patient
        information and education
    by people with CRPS 20, 36, 42, 51,
        69–70, 109–10, 115–16
    stock stories 42, 51, 109–10

Complex Regional Pain Syndrome (CRPS)
  acceptance 30, 31, 43, 64–5, 90, 106–7
  Bath CPRS centre and rehabilitation programme 27, 34, 87, 95
  and behaviour see behaviour
  and the body see body reactions
  and carers see carers
  case studies of people living with 25–91
  coping with see coping strategies
  denial of 96
  diagnosis see diagnosis of CRPS
  and feelings see feelings
  health professionals' non-recognition/ lack of understanding 27–8, 30, 33, 46, 52–3, 60–61, 66–8, 74–5
  improvement and recovery 15, 85
  internet information/searches on 20–21, 28, 40, 53, 66–7, 70, 81, 124–5
  loss with see loss
  names previously used for 16
  pain severity see pain severity
  resources 133–8
  and social life see social life
  suffering in silence 96
  support see support
  symptoms and characteristics 15–16, 20, 28–30, 38–9, 45–6, 48, 59–60, 66–7, 79, 81–2 see also pain severity
  and thoughts see thinking
  treatment see treatment of CRPS
compromise 34, 116
control 28, 32–3, 36, 41, 43
  disempowerment 52–4, 57, 67–8, 71, 74–5
  self-harming to regain 77
  sense of losing control 73, 74–5
  see also independence
coping strategies 34, 96–119
  acceptance 30, 31, 43, 64–5, 90, 106–7
  behavioural 34, 49, 62, 63–4, 90, 109–16
  with body reactions 99–102
  with feelings 84, 102–5
  hiding symptoms and pain 55, 57, 75–6, 96, 125

less effective strategies 55, 57, 96–7, 125
  Padesky and Mooney coping model 97–8, 98
  with pain 78, 83–4 see also pain relief
  of positive outlook see positive attitude
  sexual 78
  with thoughts 34, 51, 105–9
  unconscious 30
  using a range of 50–51
crisis cards 107–9, 108
CRPS see Complex Regional Pain Syndrome

daily activities 43, 63, 87–8, 111, 113–15, 114
De Mos, M. et al. 15
denial 96
desensitization 19, 126
despair 66–7
diagnosis of CRPS 16–17, 27, 33, 39, 46–7, 67, 72, 73, 86–7, 95
  and fear of worst-case scenarios 34, 40, 46, 47, 73–4, 125
  health professionals' non-recognition/ lack of understanding 27–8, 30, 33, 52–3, 60–61, 66–8, 74–5
  insensitively given 79–80
  relief at 40, 47
  without explanation 52, 53, 79–80
diary-keeping 84, 103–4
disempowerment 52–4, 57, 67–8, 71, 74–5

education, patient see patient information and education
employers 39, 41, 87
employment loss 20, 41, 70
energy levels 63, 111
  of carers 126

family
  as carers see carers
  communicating with 36, 53, 55, 70, 107
  misunderstandings 55
  therapy 70–71
fear
  of abandonment 20
  of going out 20
  and the GP–patient relationship 69
  of impact on others 75–6, 84
  of not being believed 40

and the Padesky and Mooney coping
  model 98
and paralysis 75
of people and busy places 41–2
and uncertainty 66
of what others may think 75–6
and worst-case scenarios 34, 40, 46,
  47, 73–4, 125
see also anxiety
feelings
  acknowledging and naming the
    feeling 104
  communicating 36, 115–16
  giving in to negative feelings 42
  negative feelings towards affected part
    of body 55, 60, 77, 82–3
  and the Padesky and Mooney coping
    model 98, *98*
  strategies to cope with 84, 102–5
  venting 84, 102–4
Four Pillars of Care 17–21, *17*
fresh air 102
friends
  as carers *see* carers
  loss of 35, 41
  who also have CRPS 35–6
  and work colleagues 41, 42
frustration 37, 46, 47, 55, 57, 83, 88,
  102, 123

goal setting 20, 111
Goebel, A. *et al.* 15
graded motor imagery 19
grief 35
guilt 102

hand therapy 26–7
Haydon, Virginia 110–12
helplessness, learned 57
humour 47–8, 104–5

IASP (International Association for the
  Study of Pain) 16
identity loss/change 20, 28–9, 35, 55–6,
  70
independence 62–3, 87
  loss of 20, 34–5, 87–8, 125–6
International Association for the Study of
  Pain (IASP) 16
internet 20–21, 28, 40, 53, 66–7, 70,
  81, 124–5
intimacy 20
isolation 41–2, 55, 76, 97, 118

job loss 20, 41, 70

learned helplessness 57
life grids 113–15, *114*
listening 116
loss
  experienced by carers 127–8
  of friends 35, 41
  and frustration 88 *see also* frustration
  and grief 35
  identity loss/change 20, 28–9, 35,
    55–6, 70
  of independence 20, 34–5, 62, 87–8,
    125–6
  of job 20, 41, 70
  of mobility 88–9
  and psychological help 20
medication 18, 26–7, 39, 43, 47, 48, 53,
  61, 67–8
  self-medication 74
  side effects 28
mindfulness 36, 49
mirror therapy 19, 83
mobility 88–9
monitoring 125–6

negative thoughts 20, 51, 76, 103, 117
Norton, Graham 118

occupational therapists 19

pacing 34, 63–4, 90, 110–12
Padesky, C.A. and Mooney, K.A., coping
  model 97–8, *98*
pain relief 18, 26–7, 67–8
  with orgasm 78
  side effects 28
  strategies 78, 83–4
  and swearing 103
  see also medication
pain severity 15, 28–9, 38–9, 48–9, 56,
  59, 61–2, 76, 78, 81–2, 83, 86, 90
  increased with stress 76
painting 103
panic attacks 41
patient information and education 20–21,
  30–31, 41, 56–8, 69–70
  conflicting information from health
    professionals 52–4, 67
  diagnosis of CRPS without
    explanation 52, 53, 79–80
  failure/need to check a patient's
    understanding 54, 73, 80

patient information and education *cont.*
using the internet for 20–21, 28, 40,
53, 66–7, 70, 81, 124–5
perfectionism 34
physical rehabilitation *see* rehabilitation,
physical and vocational
physiotherapy/physiotherapists 19,
60–61, 80–81, 83, 86, 127
planning 111–12
positive attitude 43–4, 65, 84, 85, 89
noting and writing down positive
things 103–4
prioritizing 111
protection 125–6
psychological interventions 19–20

Reflex Sympathy Dystrophy *see* Complex
Regional Pain Syndrome (CRPS)
rehabilitation, physical and vocational
18–19
Bath service 27, 34, 87, 95
and carers 123–4, 126–7
experiences of attending a programme
29–31, 34–5, 69
relaxation
CDs 99–100
strategies 20, 64, 99–102
responsibility 28, 125–6
and the 'blame game' 27
see also control
routines 111
RSD *see* Complex Regional Pain
Syndrome (CRPS)
rules, self-imposed 106

Samaritans 107
self-esteem, loss of 20
self-harm 77
see also suicidal thoughts
sex 78
social life
dealing with loss of 20
meeting others with CRPS 36, 50,
77–8
removing self from 41–2, 55, 76, 97,
118
stock stories 42, 51, 109–10
stress management 20
loss of means of 54
recognizing signs and triggers of stress
100
relaxation strategies 20, 64, 99–102
venting feelings 84, 102–4

suicidal thoughts 76–7, 107
leading to an attempted suicide 56, 70
support 35–6
accessing and accepting 113–15
carers *see* carers
humour as 104–5
network for carers 128
in rehabilitation 126–7
surveillance 36–7, 87
swearing 103

thinking
driven by self-imposed rules 106
habitual 105–6, 117
negative thoughts 20, 51, 76, 103,
117
and the Padesky and Mooney coping
model 98, *98*
and perfectionism 34
and positive attitude *see* positive
attitude
re-focusing 35
recognizing thoughts are just thoughts
51
strategies for dealing with thoughts
34, 51, 105–9
suicidal thoughts 56, 70, 76–7, 107
Tramadol 67–8
treatment of CRPS
anxiety over 20
and the 'blame game' 27
conflicting advice from health
professionals 67–9, 71
coping strategies *see* coping strategies
Four Pillars of Care 17–21, *17*
lack of continuity of care 53, 61
pain relief *see* pain relief
patient information *see* patient
information and education
psychological interventions 19–20
see also coping strategies; goal
setting; stress management
rehabilitation *see* rehabilitation,
physical and vocational
stress management *see* stress
management

videoing 113
visualization 99–101
vocational rehabilitation *see* rehabilitation,
physical and vocational

writing 36, 103
a diary 84, 103–4